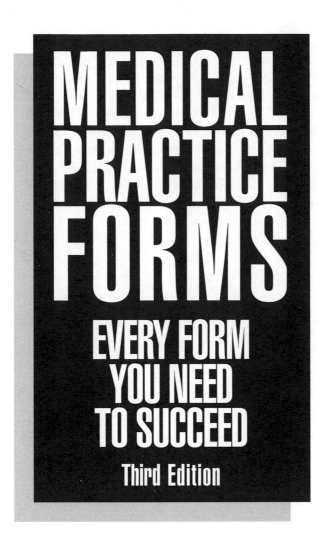

MEDICAL PRACTICE FORMS

EVERY FORM YOU NEED TO SUCCEED

Third Edition

Keith C. Borglum • Diane M. Cate

Professional Management & Marketing

Santa Rosa, California

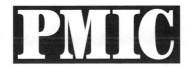

Disclaimer

This book and all the forms and information contained herein are designed to provide accurate and authoritative information on the subject matter covered. These forms are not intended for and should not be used as a substitute for specific legal, tax or other professional advice. Check the laws for your state before using any forms that have legal implications. All information contained in this guide is based on the experience of the author and the recommendations are to be considered the opinion of the author. It is sold with the understanding that neither the publisher nor author is engaged in rendering legal, medical, accounting, or other professional service in specific situations. Although prepared by professionals, this publication should not be utilized as a substitute for professional service in specific situations. If legal or medical advice is required, the services of a professional should be sought. Neither the author nor the publisher may be held liable for any misuse or misinterpretation of the guidelines in this text. All information provided is believed and intended to be reliable, but accuracy cannot be guaranteed by the author or the publisher.

MEDICAL PRACTICE FORMS: Every Form You Need to Succeed

ISBN: 1-57066-300-9

Practice Management Information Corp (PMIC)
4727 Wilshire Blvd.
Los Angeles, CA 90010
1 (800) MED-SHOP

http://www.pmiconline.com

Printed in the United States of America

TABLE OF CONTENTS

Preface

FORMS   **# of PAGES**

Administrative

Clinical

Financial

HIPAA

Insurance

Managed Care

Marketing

Personnel

Systems

PREFACE

Medical practices continue to experience significant changes. Practices of every size, from solo to academic multi-specialty integrated groups, can no longer afford inefficiency and waste. At the same time, physicians and staff face increasing burdens of paperwork.

One basic technique for improving efficiency is to organize information and paper flow. Since the largest expense in most practices is labor, any time you can save labor you will also save money and increase profits. However, the paperless office is still just a dream. Efficiency sometimes requires a certain amount of paperwork, but of a type that saves time and reduces the need for other paperwork. For example, when it is filled out by the patient and organized in an efficient manner, a comprehensive patient history form saves the physician time and eliminates the need to write in the patient chart. That same form increases the quality of care by allowing the physician time to focus on the most relevant clinical issues related to the visit. Furthermore, there is additional liability protection, since the patient filled out the information in his or her own hand—if the information is inaccurate, it is likely to be the patient's error rather than the physician's.

Well-organized administrative records save the practice business office even more time and money. They are a key to successful practice management.

The following pages contain forms, any one of which may pay for the cost of this book many times over. You are encouraged to take a hard look at each one and determine how it may fit into your practice. The forms are set up to copy directly onto your letterhead. Or, if they need to be customized to fit your practice, do it!

Instructions

The forms were developed in modern Microsoft Word® 97-98 software, which can be opened by both Windows® and Macintosh® operating systems. This format was selected after our survey indicated that virtually every physician office or household has Microsoft Word® software, or a translator. Your local print shop will also have it, as will any quick-print shop.

To use a form, copy the document from the enclosed disk(s) onto your computer desktop and customize it for your practice. You can change the size, the contents, the look, the type styles or anything you want. Please note that you are required by federal copyright law to maintain the copyright-holder mark on the document. Create a folder for your customized forms. Alternatively, you can just cut the form out of the book and photocopy it on plain paper or directly onto your letterhead. We recommend placing the original from the book, or your edited master, into a plastic sleeve for protection. Most plastic sleeves allow photocopying through the plastic. Sleeves can be obtained with spines punched for a three-hole binder, and this is a handy way to keep masters organized and stored near your copier.

Specifications

Platform	Windows® or Macintosh®
Software	1998 or later version of Microsoft Word®
Fonts	Predominantly Times Roman, Arial, Garamond and Palatino
Margins	Usually half inch top and bottom, 1" left and .75" right

If you are going to have the copy shop do the customization, just mark up a photocopy of the page from the book and take it with the disk(s) to the shop. It couldn't be easier!

A Word about Customizing and Copyright

This book and the forms in both their original form and customized to your needs are protected by federal copyright laws. You are allowed to make unlimited copies for use in your individual practice. You are not allowed to make copies for, or share the forms with, others. An individual practice is defined as under one ownership using one letterhead in one location. An easy way to keep track is that if you are using a form in more than one location, you are probably violating copyright. Just like a book, a form can be in only one place.

Consultants, MSOs, IPAs, GPWWs, academic institutions, print shops and others having need for multiple use are encouraged to call to arrange multiple-use discounts. The penalties for commercial violation of copyright are much more expensive than the cost of compliance. For multiple use discounts, call PMIC at 1-800-Med-Shop, from 9 a.m. to 5 p.m. Pacific Standard Time.

Credits and Consulting

The forms in this book were developed over a decade's consulting to over 500 medical practices, mostly in California. The authors, Keith Borglum and Diane Cate, are partners in Professional Management and Marketing in Santa Rosa, California, and are actively involved in consulting on a day-to-day basis on all the business issues facing physicians in their practices today. Their articles and opinions are widely published in many practice management periodicals, including the *AMA News, Medical Economics, Physicians' Management* and *MGMA Update.* They are or have been variously members of the National Association of Healthcare Consultants, Society of Medical Dental Management Consultants, American Medical Association's Doctors Advisory Network, American Academy of Family Physicians' Network of Consultants, ACP-ASIM Network of Consultants, the Institute of Business Appraisers, and the Professional Association of Health Care Office Managers; in addition, they are affiliate members of the Medical Group Management Association. Consulting inquiries are directed to call 1-800-79-CONSULT, or go to *www.PracticeMgmt.com* for a list of services.

Special thanks in the production of this book are given to Jill "Nimble-Fingers" Brown.

Suggestions

Suggestions and contributions for additional forms for the next edition of this book are welcome. Those submitting forms to be used in the next edition should accompany them with a letter verifying that the form is free of copyright restriction, and they will be credited by name in the book. Mail the forms to Forms Book, PMM, 3468 Piner Road, Santa Rosa, CA 95401-3954.

Administrative Forms

Introduction

When we do Practice Improvement Surveys of practices, one of the first things we do when we walk in is to take a look at the practices' method of organizing and accessing information. This can tell us a lot about what we can expect to find at every level of assessment. Well-run practices tend to have their documents in order. Poor document organization often foretells weak policies, disorganization, inadequate teamwork, ineffective management and lower profitability.

The first "form" in this section is really more of a system than a form. The Administrative Filing System is an excellent place to start because as you begin to use and modify the forms in this book, you'll need a place to put them where you can find them again. Do you have any great forms you have created? Submit them and we might put them in the next edition, and give you credit. Your form could become a national standard! See the Preface of this book for details.

ADMINISTRATIVE FILING SYSTEM

ACCOUNTING
Bank Deposit Receipts
Bank Statements (Reconciled)
Bookkeeping Forms
Bookkeeping Records
Expense Accounts
Expenses
    Answering Service and Pager
    Auto
    Building Lease
    Education and Meetings
    Equipment Purchase
    Furniture and Equipment Lease
    Insurance
    Legal and Accounting
    Loan Repayment
    Maintenance
    Medical and Drug Supplies
    Miscellaneous
    Office Supplies
    Personnel Canceled Payroll Checks
    Personnel Tax and Withholding Statements
    Petty Cash
    Postage
    Subscription and Dues
    Telephone
    Utilities
Financial Reports
    Financial goals
    Financial Projections
    Graphs
    Production and Collection Reports
    Profit and Loss Statements
Individual Patient Charge Tickets
Internal Audit Reports
Notices of Bankruptcy
Pension and Profit Sharing
Purchase Orders for Capital Expenditures

ARTICLES
Medical (by Subject)
Marketing

BROCHURES

INSTRUCTIONS
ADMINISTRATIVE FILING SYSTEM
Subject and Topic Headings

The following is a compilation of subjects considered to be standard sections for an administrative filing system as well as some of the more major topics that fall within those subjects. You may want to make additions as you come across additional subjects and topics suited to your individual practice.

Read through the list and modify it to suit your practice. Create an INDEX for your practice (easier on computer for future modification).

Type each title onto a half-inch file folder label.

Purchase adequate nine-by twelve-inch (letter size) manila file folders, third cut (three tabs across), and attach a typed label to each.

Purchase adequate file folder hangars and clear adequate file drawers for the system.

Set up the system by itself and then file your existing records into the system, writing the file name in the upper right hand corner of any document filed (see attached).

Thereafter, all documents to be filed must have an exact file name from the INDEX in the upper right-hand corner.

All persons generating filing should have their own copies of the INDEX.

When new files are created, note that on the master INDEX and periodically update all staff copies.

ADMINISTRATIVE FILING SYSTEM

CONTINUING EDUCATION
CONTRACTS AND AGREEMENTS
CORPORATION OR PARTNERSHIP
Accounting—Special
Agreements and Stockholders List
Annual Meeting—Proceedings
Annual Reports
    Worksheets
Articles of Incorporation
Board Minutes
Committee Minutes
Correspondence
    Sent
    Interoffice
    Received
Insurance

CORRESPONDENCE—Outside
Sent
Received
Interoffice

EQUIPMENT
Directions/Manuals
Inventory List with Serial and Model Numbers
Warranties with Receipts Attached

FORMS—Blank
Master Copies
Spreadsheets
Recall Tracking
Will Call Sheets

FURNITURE AND FIXTURES
INDEX TO FILING SYSTEM
INSURANCE (copies in safety deposit box)
Disability
Health
Liability and Fire
Life
Malpractice
Office Inventory (of all valuables, keep copy in safety deposit box)

INVESTMENTS

6

ADMINISTRATIVE FILING SYSTEM

LEASES
Building and Grounds
Equipment
Expired
General
Property
Vehicles

LEGAL
General
Records Retention

LICENSES AND PERMITS
Business License
DEA
General
Medical License
Hospital Privileges

MAILING LISTS

MARKETING
Ads
Logo Master
Referrer Tracking
Yellow Pages Contract

MEMBERSHIPS

OFFICE PROCEDURES MANUAL

ORGANIZATION CHART

OUTSIDE SERVICES

PERSONAL MATTERS

PERSONNEL
Applications
Individual File (by Employee), Last Name, First Name, Date of Hire
Leaves and Vacation Records
Personnel Hiring forms
Personnel Review Forms
Personnel Policies Manual

PUBLICATIONS/SUBSCRIPTIONS
Articles in Process
Articles Submitted
Articles Published
"On Hold"—to Order in Future
Subscriptions, Current

PURCHASE ORDERS

PURCHASE REQUISITIONS

REAL ESTATE RECORDS

8

ADMINISTRATIVE FILING SYSTEM

RECALL
    Audit Forms
    System Instructions
    Tracking by Month

REPORTS
    Annual
    General

RESOURCES
    Accountant
    Attorney
    Consultants
    Collections Agency
    Financial Planner
    Insurance Agents
    Labs
    Mailing Services
    Printers

SEMINARS AND WORKSHOPS
    Attended
    Pending

STATIONERY AND ENVELOPES—Master Forms and Artwork

TAXES
    City
    Federal
    State

UNEMPLOYMENT COMPENSATION

10

AFFIDAVIT TO ACCOMPANY MEDICAL RECORDS

I_____(custodian of records of patient_____)
do hereby declare:

1. I am the duly authorized custodian of the medical records of _____,
    M.D., or other qualified witness with authority to certify the records.

2. [ ] The records you seek may contain information regarding alcohol or drug abuse records, the
    results of a blood test for HIV, or information regarding certain psychiatric, mental health, or
    developmental disabilities. This information, if it exists, may be protected by special state and
    federal laws and cannot be released without specific written authorization by the patient or
    pursuant to other procedures established by law. A subpoena or general authorization for
    release of medical records is not sufficient.

    [ ] I do not have the records described in the subpoena.

    [ ] These medical records are true copies of all the records in my possession described in the
    subpoena which are allowed by law to be released.

    [ ] The records described in the subpoena and authorized by law to be released were delivered to
    _____ on _____ (date)

3. I declare under penalty of perjury that the above statements are true and correct and that this
    declaration was made at _____, on _____ (date)

Signed:_____

Print name: _____ Phone _____

ASSOCIATE PHYSICIAN/PA/FNP EVALUATION

This review is designed to provide feedback and guidance to the new physician or PA/FNP in our group to facilitate smoother integration and accelerate success. We wish to stress the importance of balance in skills in work performance.

For:_____ By: _____

Period from:_____ To:_____ Next Review: _____

A. Day-to-Day Practice	Excl.*	Good	OK	N.I.+	N/A#	Comments
1. Relationship with patients						
2. On time to office						
3. Charts, referring letters, hospital dictation on time						
4. Billing information						
5. Telephone calls effectiveness						
6. Other						
B. Practice Development						
1. Generates new patients						
2. Retains existing patients						
3. Develops referral relationships						
4. Practice marketing						
5. Suggests improvements in practice						
6. Other						
C. Practice Style						
1. Work ethic/production						
2. Utilization, cost-effectiveness, efficiency						
3. Enthusiasm						
4. Flexibility/performance under pressure						
5. Other						
D. Clinical Performance						
1. Demonstrates knowledge/skill						
2. Demonstrates diagnostic ability						
3. Proper chart documentation						
4. Patient compliance						
5. Continuing education						
6. Other						

*Excel. = Excellent
+N.I. = Needs improvement
#N/A = Not applicable.

Perform on new associates or extenders monthly for three months and then quarterly until the end of the first year at least. If you are brave, let them perform them quarterly on you too.

ASSOCIATE PHYSICIAN/PA/FNP EVALUATION

E. Interpersonal Skills	Excl.*	Good	OK	N.I.+	N/A#	Comments
1. With lay staff						
2. With referring doctors						
3. With hospital medical staff						
4. With hospital lay staff						
5. Other						
F. Miscellaneous						
1. Assistance in practice management						
2. Support of practice goals						
3. Other						

Excel.   = Excellent
+N.I.   = Needs improvement
#N/A   = Not applicable

Evaluation performed by: _____ Date: _____

Evaluation received by: _____ Date: _____

16

ASSOCIATE SPACE-SHARING CHECKLIST

Compatibility
Reference Checks Both Ways

Financial
Expense Division
        Basic Formula
        Subsidies/Deferrals/Security
        Compensation to Doctor for Administration
        Formula for Shared Purchases in Future
        Excluded Income/Expenses
        When Paid/Reserve/Deposit
        Disability/Death Obligations
Equity Balancing
Document Equity Contributions Ongoing
Buy-in/Pay-out Formula
Accountability/Audit Rights
Compensation for Call Coverage/Nonmember Plans
Linked Entity Retirement Plan Issues
Sublet Full Services
Practice Purchase Rights in Death/Disability/Other
Hospital Financial Assistance

Governance and Decision Making
Structure
Length/Duration
Minority Rights
Disagreements/Arbitration
Reporting/Meetings
Relatives in Practice
Management Responsibilities
Restrictive Covenants

Systems
Access to Office/Hours
Access to Personal Space
Personnel
        Handbook
        Needs
        Job Descriptions
        Supervisor Behavior and Risks
Call/Privileges
Patient Distribution
Phone Numbers
Fee Schedules
Malpractice Insurance
Training Schedule for New Doctor in Office Systems
Practice Promotion

Use this to set up a new agreement or evaluate an existing one.

HOW TO CHOOSE A PRACTICE MANAGEMENT CONSULTANT

What do I want them to achieve? _____

Is this a service they provide? _____

How long have they been in business? _____

What types of practices do they consult to most often? _____

Do they provide an interview at no charge? _____

Is the person I meet the person I will work with? _____

What is his or her background? _____

What are his or her strengths and weaknesses? _____

Are there backup experts with other strengths? _____

What are references can he or she provide personally? _____

Do I like this person? Can I work with him or her? _____

What references does the company have? _____

Does its contract have specific goals for my practice? _____

How much time will be provided? _____

Where? _____

What reports will be provided? _____

What are the fees? _____

Do they sell anything or take commissions on anything? _____

Have I been honest and open in explaining my needs and concerns? _____

Questions for references:

Would you use this consultant again? _____

What were his or her strengths and weaknesses? _____

Did the results warrant the costs? _____

Over 360 types of management consultants are listed in the directory of the Professional and Technical Consultants Association. Very few specialize in health care practices. A good management consultant can bring a fresh, unbiased perspective to viewing the strengths and weaknesses of your practice. According to a *Medical Economics* poll, "more than 80% of doctors who have used practice management consultants are tickled pink by the job they did."

INVENTORY CONTROL SYSTEM

Item_____
Supplier _____
Last price paid per unit _____
Buying cycle _____ Ordering lag time _____
Order amount _____ Bundle amount _____

Item_____
Supplier _____
Last price paid per unit _____
Buying cycle _____ Ordering lag time _____
Order amount _____ Bundle amount _____

Item_____
Supplier _____
Last price paid per unit _____
Buying cycle _____ Ordering lag time _____
Order amount _____ Bundle amount _____

Item_____ _____
Supplier _____
Last price paid per unit _____
Buying cycle _____ Ordering lag time _____
Order amount _____ Bundle amount _____

Item_____
Supplier _____
Last price paid per unit _____
Buying cycle _____ Ordering lag time _____
Order amount _____ Bundle amount _____

Item_____
Supplier _____
Last price paid per unit _____
Buying cycle _____ Ordering lag time _____
Order amount _____ Bundle amount _____

Item_____
Supplier _____
Last price paid per unit _____
Buying cycle _____ Ordering lag time _____
Order amount _____ Bundle amount _____

Item_____
Supplier _____
Last price paid per unit _____
Buying cycle _____ Ordering lag time _____
Order amount _____ Bundle amount _____

Inventory Control System

- Determine the buying cycle (weekly, monthly, quarterly, etc.) for each supply item.

- Determine the amounts used during the buying cycle.

- Determine the ordering lag time and bundle (wrap, box, band with string, etc.) enough for the ordering lag time. (This is your reserve bundle.)

- Tag the bundle as follows:

We buy widgets in 100-unit quantities for discount, and they last us about 2 months. Ordering plus delivery takes 2 weeks.

- When you are down to your reserve bundle, drop the tag in a special envelope or basket. Give the tags to the supply clerk weekly for ordering.

- Reattach the tag to the new bundle when the order is received.

PATIENT COUNT PER DAY ACHIEVEMENT

Date	Day M-F	Doctors/Providers											
													Goal / day
1													Notes
2													
3													
4													
5													
6													
7													
8													
9													
10													
11													
12													
13													
14													
15													
16													
17													
18													
19													
20													
21													
22													
23													
24													
25													
26													
27													
28													
29													
30													
													Total/month

Tracking patient encounters is as important as tracking dollars.

PATIENT HEALTH HISTORY UPDATE

Patient Health History Update

Date _____

NAME _____

CURRENT ADDRESS _____

CURRENT PHONE NO. Home _____ Work _____

Any changes in insurance coverage? ☐ Yes   ☐ No   ☐ N/A
If yes, please give benefits card to receptionist.

Since your last visit with us, have you:

1. Had any surgery? If so, what?
   ☐ No
   ☐ Yes, please list _____

2. Had any health problems diagnosed? If so, what?
   ☐ No
   ☐ Yes, please list _____

3. Any change in your medications?
   ☐ No
   ☐ Yes, please list _____
4. Contracted or been exposed to hepatitis?
   ☐ No
   ☐ Yes, please list type _____

5. Contracted or been exposed to HIV (AIDS virus)?
   ☐ No
   ☐ Yes

6. If female, are you pregnant?
   ☐ No
   ☐ Yes

7. Any other health problems we should know about?
   ☐ No
   ☐ Yes, please list _____

Cut and paste two forms horizontally on one page and print. Give to every return patient.

PATIENT REGISTRATION

Welcome to our office. We are committed to providing the best, most comprehensive care possible. We encourage you to ask questions. Please assist us by providing the following information. All information is confidential and is released only with your consent. <u>Please fill in the blanks below the line.</u>

Patient Name	Today's Date	Date of Birth	Sex	Age

Parent if Patient is a Minor

Patient's Social Security Number	California Driver's License No.

Home Address	City	State	Zip

Mailing Address if Different	City	State	Zip

Home Telephone Number	Work Telephone Number

Occupation	Employer's Name

Employer's Address	City	State	Zip

Spouse Name	Employer

Other Physician's Name

Whom May We Thank for Referring You to Our Practice?

NOTIFY IN CASE OF EMERGENCY

Name	Relationship

Address	City	State	Zip

Home Telephone	Work Telephone

Nearest Relative (not living with your)

Home Telephone	Work Telephone

FINANCIAL INFORMATION: PERSON RESPONSIBLE FOR FEES

Name	Telephone

Address	City	State	Zip

Insurance Company	Claim Address

Subscriber's Name	Subscriber's Date of Birth	Subscriber's SSN#.

Insurance ID No.:
Secondary Insurance	Claim Address

Subscriber's Name	Subscriber's Date of Birth	Subscriber's SSN#

Were You Injured on the Job? YES NO	Have you Informed Your Employer? YES NO
Date of Original Injury:	
Worker's Compensation Carrier Name	Address

Please Read Our Financial Policy Statement and Agreement on Reverse

A patient registration form requiring financial policies to be printed on the back.

PATIENT SIGN-IN SHEET

		Please Sign In		
Date	Time In	Patient Name—Please Print	Appt. Time	

The above should be used to have patients sign in. This helps with "internal security" and provides documentation on time management.

PHONE NURSE LOG

Patient	Date	Time	Question/Response	Initials

31

ROUTING SLIPS

ROUTING SLIP

Date _____

Item: _____

Route to: _____

_____

_____

_____

_____

_____

_____

_____

_____

_____

When finished, cross out your name and pass on.

ROUTING SLIP

Date _____

Item: _____

Route to: _____

_____

_____

_____

_____

_____

_____

_____

_____

_____

When finished, cross out your name and pass on.

ROUTING SLIP

Date _____

Item: _____

Route to: _____

_____

_____

_____

_____

_____

_____

_____

_____

_____

When finished, cross out your name and pass on.

ROUTING SLIP

Date _____

Item: _____

Route to: _____

_____

_____

_____

_____

_____

_____

_____

_____

_____

When finished, cross out your name and pass on.

Cut and paste, print and pad.

SIGNATURE LOG

A copy of this log shall be maintained in the practice administrative files. The log should be updated to reflect the current signature and initials of each individual making entries into patient records.

Physician/Employee   Employee Dates

_____   _____   From_____   To_____
Full Name, Title   Initials

_____   _____
Signature   Date   Initials

_____   _____   From_____   To _____
Full Name, Title   Initials

_____   _____
Signature   Date   Initials

_____   _____   From_____   To_____
Full Name, Title   Initials

_____   _____
Signature   Date   Initials

_____   _____   From _____   To _____
Full Name, Title   Initials

_____   _____
Signature   Date   Initials

_____   _____   From _____   To _____
Full Name, Title   Initials

_____   _____
Signature   Date   Initials

A helpful form when the attorneys come knocking.

WEEKLY COMPUTER BACKUP LOG

Date	Who	Date Disk Title	Date	Who	Data Disk Title

MEDICAL RECORD COMPLIANCE EVALUATION

SITE ADDRESS

REPORT RECEIVED BY:

PHYSICIAN NAME: _____ ID# _____

EVALUATOR: _____ PT ID: _____

SPECIALTY: _____

DATE: _____ SIGNATURE: _____

	Patient #1	Patient #2	Patient #3	Patient #4	Patient #5
	Y/N/NA	Y/N/NA	Y/N/NA	Y/N/NA	Y/N/NA
1. Do all pages contain patient's name?					
2. Is there personal data?					
3. Are all entries signed and identified by author?					
4. Are all entries dated?					
5. Are all entries legible?					
6. Is there a problem list in use?					
7. Are allergies and adverse reactions noted and flagged?					
8. Is there a current medical history and physical exam in the record?					
9. Are there progress notes with vital signs for each visit?					
10. Are lab and other studies ordered and filed appropriately?					
11. Are working diagnoses consistent with findings?					
12. Are plans of action/treatment consistent with diagnosis?					
13. Is there a date for return visit or other follow-up plan for each encounter?					
14. Are problems from previous visits addressed?					
15. Is there evidence of appropriate use of specialists?					
16. Is there evidence of continuity and coordination of care between PCP and specialists?					
17. Do consultant summaries, lab and imaging results reflect PCP review (and initialed)?					
18. Does the care appear to be medically appropriate?					
19. Is there a completed immunization record?					
20. Are preventive services appropriately used?					
21. Is there documentation of smoking habits and history of alcohol use or substance abuse?					
22. Evidence of patient education/counseling for:					
A. Heart disease risk factors? (See key)	N N/A A1 A2 A3 A4 A5	N N/A A1 A2 A3 A4 A5	N N/A A1 A2 A3 A4 A5	N N/A A1 A2 A3 A4 A5	N N/A A1 A2 A3 A4 A5
B. Prevention of motor vehicle injury?					
C. Sexually transmitted disease screening and prevention?					
D. HIV screening and prevention?					
E. Alcoholism screening and prevention?					
F. Drug abuse screening and prevention?					

KEY: For question 22-A, circle one of the following for "Y" response on each patient chart: A1=smoking, A2=cholesterol, A3=exercise, A4=hypertension, A5=general diet

©2003 Professional Management & Marketing

DRUG INVENTORY LOG

Date	Drug Name	Amount Removed/Added	By	Confirmed

42

EMERGENCY KIT INSPECTION LOG

Emergency Kit Inspection Log

Date: _____

By location: _____

Supplies stocked: _____

Supplies current: _____

Instruments stocked: _____

Equipment works: _____

Equipment current: _____

Items replaced: _____

Emergency Kit Inspection Log

Date: _____

By location: _____

Supplies stocked: _____

Supplies current: _____

Instruments stocked: _____

Equipment works: _____

Equipment current: _____

Items replaced: _____

Emergency Kit Inspection Log

Date: _____

By location: _____

Supplies stocked: _____

Supplies current: _____

Instruments stocked: _____

Equipment works: _____

Equipment current: _____

Items replaced: _____

44

EXAM ROOM INVENTORY INSPECTION LOG

Date	Exam Room #	Supplies Stocked & Current	Instruments Stocked	Equipment Works	Notes

NEW PATIENT FLOW SHEET

Today's Date: _____

Appointment

- ◆ Patient Name   _____
- ◆ Parent Name   _____
- ◆ Referred By   _____
- ◆ Forms Sent   _____
- ◆ Forms Rcvd. Complete   _____
- ◆ Appointment Date & Time   _____

Check In

- ◆ Shown New Patient Video   _____
- ◆ Brochure & Card Given   _____
- ◆ Office Tour/Intros Done   _____

Check Out

- ◆ Any Questions Need Answering   _____
- ◆ Confirm H & P Up-to-date   _____
- ◆ Next Appointment Made   _____
- ◆ Letter to Patient Mailed   _____
- ◆ Referrer Thank You Sent   _____

Office Manager Approval   _____

48

MANAGED CARE SPECIALIST REVIEW WORKSHEET

MANAGED CARE SPECIALIST REVIEW WORKSHEET

Specialty _____
Review (initials or code) _____
Community _____

Rate 1 – 5:
1=unacceptable, 2=below average, 3=average, 4=good, 5=excellent

	Physicians & Location										
1. **Quality of Care** — How is their care relative to same specialty MDs in your community?											
2. **Peer Respect** — How respected is this MD among other same specialty MDs?											
3. **General Respect** — How respected is this MD among all MDs in your community?											
4. **Patient Satisfaction** — How satisfied have patients been with care provided by this specialist?											
5. **Availability** — How easy is it to get a patient in to see this specialist?											
6. **Cooperativeness** — How well do they work with you on issues related to patients?											
7. **Communication** — How good is this person at providing you information about your patients?											
8. **Location** — How convenient is their location to your patients?											
9. **Office Setting** — Is their office modern, attractive and in an area perceived as safe after dark?											
10. **Cost Containment** — How interested are they in controlling healthcare costs?											
11. **Flexibility** — How adaptable do you think this MD would be to changes required by managed care?											
12. **Group** — If this MD is in a group, please rate your overall impression of the rest of the group.											
13. **Competition** — Rate freedom from involvement in competing entities (5 is free, 1 is wholly encumbered).											
14. **Special Problems** — Please note and rate any additional problems or issues that might affect their ability to manage care.											
TOTAL POINTS											
RATING											

Total points ÷ by (number of categories rate x 5) = percent
Ex: 36 points ÷ (11 categories rate x 5) = 65.4% rating.
Rating: The higher the percentage, the more attractive the physician.

*Clinical Forms*_____

Introduction

There are two major reasons for improving the paperwork related to clinical care. The first is to improve quality of care to the patient, and the second is to reduce legal liability. The more organized the approach to care, the less likely that an omission will occur by doctor or staff. None of our memories is perfect and we can all use help.

It would be impossible to include forms for every one of the more than 200 recognized medical specialties. We have included representative samples for you to consider modifying to your needs.

BRIEF HISTORY

In an effort to serve you better, we request that you provide us with the following information. We need this information to give you the best care and treatment possible. All information is held strictly confidential and is released only with your written consent.

Last Name:	First:	Age:	Sex:	Doctor Notes _please do not write in this area_

Presenting Problem or Proposed Surgery:

ILLNESS/INJURY: Please check if you have ever had:

Yes	No		Yes	No	
		High blood pressure			Kidney Stones
		Diabetes			Abdominal bleeding
		Peptic ulcers			Diverticulosis
		Heart attack			Thyroid problem
		Chest pain/tightness			Lung problems/asthma
		History of heart murmur			Shortness of breath
		Stroke			Accidents/broken bones (list)
		Cancer			
		Hepatitis			
		Yellow jaundice			
		Gallstones			

OPERATIONS: List names and dates of all operations you have had ☐ None

Year	Name of Operation	Type of Anesthetic, if Known	Complications

Have you ever had a blood transfusion? ☐ Yes   ☐ No   Date: _____

List any hospital admissions or medical conditions not list above:

FEMALES ONLY: Are you pregnant? ☐ Yes   ☐ No

DRUGS: Please list all drugs you take and their dosages. ☐ None

Drug	Dosage	Drug	Dosage

ALLERGIES: Please list type and reaction ☐ None

Name of Drug	Reaction	Name of Drug	Reaction

Do you now use tobacco? ☐ Yes   ☐ No   Day # Yrs ___ /____

Have you ever used tobacco? ☐ Yes   ☐ No   Yrs Quit _____

Do you drink alcohol? ☐ Yes   ☐ No   Day # Yrs ___ /____

Have you ever used alcohol? ☐ Yes   ☐ No   Yrs Quit _____

Type: _____

The above information is true and accurate.

Patient Signature (parent if patient is a minor)_____

Typically used for a brief new managed care visit, for a brief specialist visitor, or before a simple referred procedure.

BRIEF VISIT RECORD

Patient:

Date: Time in: Provider:

Purpose of Visit:

s/o/a/p:

RX/Immunizations   Time out:

Patient:

Date: Time in: Provider:

Purpose of Visit:

s/o/a/p:

RX/Immunizations   Time out:

Patient:

Date: Time in: Provider:

Purpose of Visit:

s/o/a/p:

RX/Immunizations   Time out:

Use as a page in a patient chart for progress notes.

CARDIOLOGY REFERRAL REQUEST

CARDIOLOGY REFERRAL REQUEST

Date _____

Patient Name _____

Referring Physician: _____

History _____

_____

_____

SERVICES REQUESTED

_____ Consultation   _____ Brief Opinion

_____ 12-Lead Electrocardiogram and Interpretation

_____ Exercise Stress Test   _____ Pacemaker check

_____ Pacemaker Check with Follow-up

_____ 24-Hour Holter Monitor

_____ M-Mode/2D Echocardiogram

_____ Echocardiogram with Doppler

_____ Noninvasive Peripheral Vascular Study

            _____ Arterial   _____ Venous

APPOINTMENT

Date: _____ Time _____

CHART SETUP

Left	Right
Top Down *Newest on Top*	*Top Down* *Newest On Top*
Summary Sheet Dictation	Insurance Information Path Reports Lab Reports X-Ray Reports Op Reports Discharge Summaries H+Ps Letters from/to Doctors

Typical setup for patient chart. Post in filing and chart setup area.

CONSULTATION/NEUROLOGICAL

Appointment Time: _____ Date: _____

Your first appointment will consist of one of the following:

☐ **Consultation**
The neurologist will review your medical history and evaluate the symptoms involving your nervous system. He or she will then assess the various parts of your nervous system by testing strength, sensation, coordination, reflexes, and mental and language function. As necessary, a general physical examination is performed to investigate possible medical conditions affecting your nervous system. further tests, if needed, are usually scheduled for another visit.

Testing and Studies
When scheduling one of the following, you will be sent an explanation of the procedures and any instructions or preparation necessary to your visit.

☐ **NCT (nerve conduction study)**
measures any blocking or slowing of nerve conduction

☐ **EMG (electromyography)**
tests for disorders of muscles or nerves connected to the muscles

☐ **EEG (electroencephalography)**
tests for disturbances or injuries related to the brain

☐ **BIOFEEDBACK**
a technique to control headache, backache, stress, chronic pain, and other disorders

☐ **ENG (electronystagmography)**
tests for disorders related to the ear, nerve to the ear, and central portion of the brain

☐ **TNS (transcutaneous nerve stimulator)**
a device for relieving pain without medication

Instructions to Patient

Your appointment time is reserved exclusively for you. Please make every effort to be on time. Please give at least 24 hour's notice if a change is needed. You will receive additional instructions and information in the mail prior to your appointment.

If this is a work-related injury, bring:
- Your insurance company name
- Case number and date of injury
- Evidence of insurance and company authorization
- Name & phone number of authorizing claims person

If You Have Any Questions, Please Call Us at _____

Format can be modified for any specialty or for a procedure visit in practice.

DIABETES FLOW SHEET

Patient: _____

Date	Wt/Ht	Blood Sugar	BP	GLUC/ KET	UA PRO	Hb AIC	Medication Insulin/Oral

Visits: _____ Diet Order: _____

Use for every patient visit.

DIABETES HEALTH MAINTENANCE RECORD

Patient: _____

	Years									
	20___	20___	20___	20___	20___	20___	20___	20___	20___	20___
Pap/Pelvic/Breast and/or Rectal Exam										
Mammogram Yearly										
Dietary Clinic Yearly										
Flu Vaccine Yearly										
Serum Creatinine Yearly										
U/A for Protein Yearly										
Ophthalmology Exam Yearly										
Screening for Neuropathy Yearly										
CBC Every 3 Years										
ECG/CXR Every 5 Years										
Td Booster Every 10 Years										
Pneumovax 1 Dose Only										
PPD Screening and as Indicated										
Serology Screening and as Indicated										
Hb, A1, C										
Others										

GI CONSULT OR FLEXIBLE SIGMOIDOSCOPY

Appointment Time: _____ Date: _____

Your first appointment will consist of one of the following:

☐ **Consultation**

This visit will not involve any technical procedures or tests. No special diet or preparation is needed. The doctor will take a detailed history and perform a physical examination, then discuss your entire problem in detail with you. He or she will arrange any further testing or treatment necessary. Please allow 90 minutes for this visit.

☐ **Consultation with Flexible Sigmoidoscopy**

This visit will involve a consultation as above, plus an exam consisting of insertion of a thin, flexible instrument into the rectum and large bowel to inspect for any possible irregularities. Please call the office prior to your appointment to determine if any bowel preparation will be required before your examination. Please allow 2 hours for this visit.

☐ **Screening Flexible Sigmoidoscopy**

This visit will consist of insertion, of a thin, flexible instrument into the rectum and large bowel to inspect for any possible irregularities. Preparation will be necessary so that the procedure can be performed comfortably and safely. The following will be necessary:

(1) Clear liquid diet the day before the procedure. Clear liquids include broths, juices (such as apple), gelatin, etc.

(2) Magnesium citrate, one bottle, early the afternoon before the procedure.

(3) Two fleet's enemas to be taken one hour apart the morning of the procedure. Follow the instructions on the enema box. Please allow one hour for the visit.

☐ **Other/Notes:** _____

_____

_____

_____

Instructions to Patient

Please allow at least 1½ hours for your first appointment. Your appointment time is reserved exclusively for you. We make every effort to be on time. Please give *at least* 24 hours' notice if a change is needed

Payment and Insurance

Please be prepared to pay for your visit at the time of the appointment. We will be happy to help you with any paperwork. We do accept Medicare assignment and most insurance programs. If you have private insurance, please bring your benefits booklet with you. We offer you a 5% bookkeeping discount for full payment at the time of service. If you are a member of a prepaid health plan and have payment questions or if you have any other questions, please call us at _____

Format can be modified for any specialty or for a procedure visit in practice.

GYN EXAM / PROCEDURE   □ normal

Name: _____ Age: _____ Today's Date _____

DA: _____ Med: _____

Complaint/Reasons for Visit: _____

Objective:

Height: _____ Weight: _____ BP: _____ Last Menstrual Period: _____

General: _____

Thyroid: □ / _____

HEENT: □ / _____

Breasts: □ / _____

Axillae: □ / _____

Heart: □ / _____

Lungs: □ / _____

Abdomen: □ / _____

FP method _____ Date Begun _____

TAB _____ SA _____

Pelvic:

External Genitalia: □ / _____

BUS: □ / _____

Vagina: □ / _____

Cervix: □ / _____ Consistency_____

Uterus: Size: □ / _____

            Position: _____

            Tenderness: _____

Adnexae: □ / _____

Rectal: □ / _____

Extremities: □ / _____

Other: None   □ / _____

Procedures:

Pap: _____ GC: _____ Wet Mount: _____

Chlamydia: _____ Other: _____

Pregnancy Test: _____

Urinalysis: _____ Glucose: _____ Protein: _____

_____ Other _____

Assessment: _____

_____

Plan: _____

_____

HEALTH HISTORY SHEET

Welcome to our practice! To provide you with the best, most comprehensive care possible, we request that you provide the following information. All information is held strictly confidential and is released only with your written permission.

Last Name:	First:		Age:	Sex:	Doctor Notes *please do not write in this area*
Presenting Problem or Proposed Surgery:					
Have you or any blood relative had:					

	Yes	No	Who	Year
Allergies, asthma, hay fever				
Anemia				
Alcoholism				
Arthritis				
Bleeding problems				
Birth defects				
Cancer				
Emphysema				
Epilepsy or seizures				
Heart Trouble				
Mental illness				
Migraine headaches				
Rheumatic fever				
Stroke				
Suicide				
Thyroid disease/goiter				
Tuberculosis				
Ulcers				
Venereal disease				
Osteoporosis				
Glaucoma				
Gallstones				

Have you ever been turned down for military, job, insurance? ☐ Yes ☐ No

Names of Other Present MDs Last Visit	Childhood Immunizations	Year
	Tetanus	
	Childhood Diphtheria	
	Childhood Polio	
	Pneumovax	
	Flu Shot	
	Last TB Test	
	TB: ☐ Positive ☐ Negative	

ALLERGIES: Please list type and reaction ☐ NONE

Name of Drug/Item	Reaction	Name of Drug/Item	Reaction

Regular health history form for a primary care physician patient.

HEALTH HISTORY SHEET

Patient Name: _____

MEDICATIONS						Doctor Notes *do not write in this area*
Have you EVER TAKEN:	Yes	No	Year	How Long?	Brand/Descr/Dose	
Blood pressure pills						
Cortisone/steroids						
Diet pills						
Diabetes pills						
Thyroid pills						
Tranquilizers						
Water pills						
Are you NOW taking:						
Antacids						
Aspirin						
Antibiotics						
Birth control pills						
Blood thinner pills						
Laxatives						
Pain pills						
Sleeping pills						
Vitamins						
OTHER *Please list*						

OB/GYN HISTORY	Date or no. if requested	Yes	No
Date of last menstrual period:			
Are your menses irregular?			
No. of days between periods			
No. of days periods last			
Spotting between periods?			
Do you forget to do self breast exams monthly?			
Are you pregnant			
No. of pregnancies			
Date of last pregnancy			
No. of live births			
No. of abortions or miscarriages			
Date of last Pap smear			
Was it abnormal?			
Have you ever had any other abnormal Pap?			
Are you currently using contraception?			
Type of contraception			
Types of contraceptives used in past			
Did your mother take DES during her pregnancy?			
Over 1 year since last mammogram? If yes, date:			

SURGICAL HISTORY: Name of.Operation	Date	Complications

Have you ever had bleeding problems?   ☐ Yes   ☐ No
Have you ever had a blood transfusion?   ☐ Yes   ☐ No Date:_____

MAJOR ILLNESS OR INJURY: list any illness or injury requiring hospitalization, prolonged care, or use of medication. Include approximate date._____
_____
_____

73   ©2003 Professional Management & Marketing

74

HEALTH HISTORY SHEET

Patient Name: _____

PERSONAL HABITS/RISK FACTORS	Yes	No	Answers	Doctor Notes *please do no write in this area*
Do you smoke or chew tobacco?			No. packs/day:	
Have you ever smoked in the past?			Date started:	
			Date stopped:	
Do you often miss 3 meals/day?				
Do you eat snacks regularly?				
Do you have an eating problem?				
Any diet preferences/restrictions?				
Type				
Dietary habits			Frequency or No.:	
Low fat				
No. servings/day vegetables/fruits				
No. servings/day grains				
No. times/week you eat red meat				
No. servings/day dairy				
No. caffeine drinks/day				
Ave. alcoholic drinks/day				
No. times "drunk"/year				
Ever had a drinking problem?				
Ever had a drug problem?				
Every used intravenous drugs?			Date last used:	
Do you ever not use seat belts?				
No. hours sleep/day				
Highest grade level achieved				
Do you not know how to swim?				
Do you not exercise regularly?				
What exercise do you do?				
How often/week?			Duration:	
What do you do to relieve stress?				
Any pets?				
Any hobbies?				
Occupation:				
Do you hate your job?				
Is your job a risk to your health?				
If yes (in any way), please explain:				

SOCIAL HISTORY	Do you have children?
Are you: ☐ Married	☐ Yes ☐ No
☐ Divorced ☐ Single	If yes, please list No. & age(s)
☐ Widowed ☐ Living with "signif. other"	

SEXUAL HISTORY	Yes	No	Sexual partners in past year:
Are you sexually active?			No. men
Is sex unsatisfactory in any way?			No. women
History of Chlamydia?			No. unprotected
Gonorrhea?			AIDS, cont'd
Venereal warts?			Would you like to have a test?
Are you concerned about AIDS?			☐ Yes ☐ No

If there are any special concerns you would like to discuss with the doctor, please continue on the reverse of this sheet. Thank you for providing us with this important information.

IMMUNIZATION HISTORY RECORD

Patient: _____ Birthdate: _____

Immunization	Date	Dose	Site	Manufacturer and Lot Number	Initial	Comments/ Reactions
Diphtheria Tetanus Pertussis (note if DT)						
Tetanus Diphtheria (adult Td)						
Polio						
Measles, Mumps, Rubella						
Measles						
Haemophilus influenzae b						
Hepatitis B						
Gamma Globulin						
Tetanus Toxoid						
Flu Type						
Others						
Tuberculin						

INSTRUCTIONS FOR OUTPATIENT SURGERY

We would like to thank you for scheduling your surgery with Dr. _____ and want to provide you with some important information. Our aim is to keep you informed, comfortable, and confident regarding your outpatient surgery.

LAB TESTING REQUIRED: ☐ Yes ☐ No

LOCATION: ☐ (_____) Hospital ☐ Other

TIME OF SURGERY: Day: _____ Date: _____ Between _____ and _____*

*The time will be confirmed prior to the day of surgery.

ANESTHESIOLOGIST: _____

ASSISTANT SURGEON: _____

ESTIMATED PROFESSIONAL FEE of Dr. _____

Includes all your care on the day of the operation both in and out of the operating room and uncomplicated postop care for _____ days.

ANESTHESIA (Checked box indicates the type you will receive)

  ☐ A. General Anesthesia
        Adults: No smoking after midnight before operation
                  No food or drink (even water) after midnight.
        Infants: No food or drink six hours before operation, except water.

  ☐ B. Local Anesthesia
        No food or drink two hours before operation for adults and children.
        Minors: Signature of at least one parent is required. This may be done
                  at any time prior to the surgery.

All patients must be accompanied by a responsible adult during the entire stay at the hospital.

No patient should drive him/herself home from the hospital under any circumstances.

A nurse will call you the day before your surgery, and an anesthesiologist may also call. If their instructions differ from these printed instructions, disregard the printed instruction that is inconsistent with the verbal ones given you. If you have any concerns regarding instructions, please feel free to call Dr. _____ at _____. Please note: This form need not be taken to the hospital. It is for your information only.

To insure comprehensive follow-up to your surgery, your postoperative appointment at our office is scheduled for: _____.

Our commitment is to provide you with the best, most comprehensive professional care possible. Thank you for being a member of our family of patients.

The more written information you provide the patient, the fewer phone calls you will receive.

INSTRUCTIONS FOR SURGERY WITH OVERNIGHT STAY

We would like to thank you for scheduling with Dr. _____

and want to provide you with some important information. Our goal is to keep you

informed, comfortable, and confident regarding your surgery.

Name of Hospital: ☐ _____ ☐ Other _____

Address: _____

Type of Surgery: _____

Date of Surgery: _____

Name of Anesthesiologists: _____

Name of Assistant(s): _____

Be sure to enter the hospital at: _____

in order for the lab to perform the necessary tests.

Wear loose comfortable clothing and bring bed clothing if you so desire. Usual necessities

are toothbrush and toothpaste, comb or brush, cosmetics, and reading material. For your

comfort, we also recommend you bring a Walkman personal radio with headphones, and

soft earplugs for sleeping.

If you have any questions regarding the above procedures, please do not hesitate to call at

(____) _____ for assistance. We want you to be as comfortable as possible

during your hospital stay.

Thank you.

The more you can provide the patient in writing, the better.

LAB REPORT

Dear: Date:

The report of your test/records is marked below. Only the items checked or circled apply to you. Please read the entire page carefully. Please call if you have any questions.

- ☐ BLOOD PRESSURE: Checks were _____normal _____abnormal (see below)
- ☐ BLOOD TESTS: A copy of the results is/is not enclosed. (an explanation of the tests is on the back of this sheet.)
- ☐ All blood tests were normal for your age, sex, and therapy.
- ☐ The blood test(s) listed here or circled on back side of this sheet were abnormal_____(see below)
- ☐ _____ BLOOD LEVELS were:
    - ☐ normal—continue current dose.   ☐ abnormal (see below)
- ☐ CHOLESTEROL: (See back of sheet for interpretation)
- ☐ Total cholesterol now is _____, was _____
- ☐ LDL "bad" cholesterol now is _____, was _____
- ☐ HDL "good" cholesterol now is _____, was _____
- ☐ Triglyceride level now is _____, was _____
- ☐ Results on lab sheet enclosed.
- ☐ Please start low-fat diet plan, which is enclosed.
- ☐ X-RAYS: Your _____x-rays were:
    - ☐ normal   ☐ abnormal (see below)
- ☐ BREAST X-RAYS: Results were:
    - ☐ normal—please repeat in _____years   ☐ abnormal (see below)
- ☐ STOOL TEST for blood was:
    - ☐ normal—please repeat in _____years   ☐ abnormal (see below)
- ☐ ECG (heart tracing): Results were:
    - ☐ normal   ☐ abnormal (see below)
- ☐ OLD RECORDS were reviewed
    - ☐ normal   ☐ (see below)
    - PAP SMEAR was:
    - ☐ normal—please repeat in _____years   ☐ abnormal (see below)
- ☐ RECOMMENDATIONS:
    - ☐ Continue current medical therapy
    - ☐ Please call office soon to schedule an appointment for the first available time.
        Please follow up in _____. Please call several weeks ahead to schedule the appointment.
    - ☐ Please call:
    - ☐ to report how you are doing.
    - ☐ if you are still having problems.

Comment:_____

_____

....

LAB SLIP
(Cut on dotted line and bring with you to the lab.)

- ☐ Repeat test listed below in _____ .
- ☐ May eat before test.
- ☐ Only water for 12 hours before test. Take your medicine at usual time but hold diabetic medicine until you eat.

Tests _____ DX_____ PLEASE SEND RESULTS TO: NAME, M.D.

(address and phone number)

Recommend that the patient keep copies of lab reports in his or her personal medical file.

LAB REPORT

EXPLANATION OF BLOOD TESTS: The following is a general guide to the meaning of blood tests; how the results apply to you should be discussed with your doctor. Tests that are circled are abnormal. Tests that are crossed off should be ignored. Please talk to your doctor is you have questions about these results.

TEST NAME	COMMENTS
glucose	blood sugar level for diabetes
sodium, potassium, chloride, CO_2	blood minerals and acid balance
uric acid	test for gout
calcium phosphorus	bone minerals
albumin, globulin	body proteins for nutrition
bilirubin, gamma-GT, SBOT, SGPT	liver test
LDH	muscle and organs
iron, TIBC, % saturation, ferritin	body iron level
total cholesterol	normal less than 200; borderline 200-400
HDL cholesterol	measure of "good protective" cholesterol, which reduces the risk of heart disease; the higher, the better (prefer over 50)
LDL cholesterol	measure of "bad" cholesterol, which increases the risks of heart disease; the lower, the better (prefer under 130)
Triglycerides	a different blood fat
T_4, T_3RU, T_7, FTI, TSH	thyroid gland tests
wbc—white blood count	cells that fight infection
hemoglobin, hematocrit	checks for anemia
platelet count	cells that help stop bleeding
sed rate	measures level of or irritation of body

MAMMOGRAPHY REFERRAL

Early Detection of Breast Cancer Can Save Your Life.

PHYSICIAN REFERRAL FORM

Name _____ Date _____

_____ Mammography: _____ Bilateral _____ Unilateral, R-L

_____ Instruction in Breast Self-Examination

Indications _____

Higher Risk Factors

☐ Age over 50
☐ Personal and/or family
History of breast cancer
☐ Palpable breast mass
☐ Epithelial hyperplasia
☐ Age at menarche under 14
☐ Age at menopause over 55
☐ Personal history of uterine, ovarian, or colon cancer

_____
Physician's signature

An appointment scheduled for _____ a.m./p.m.

on _____

(Enter referring doctor information here)

Early Detection of Breast Cancer Can Save Your Life

PHYSICIAN REFERRAL FORM

Name _____ Date _____

_____ Mammography: _____ Bilateral _____ Unilateral, R-L

_____ Instruction in Breast Self-Examination

Indications _____

Higher Risk Factors

☐ Age over 50
☐ Personal and/or family
History of breast cancer
☐ Palpable breast mass
☐ Epithelial hyperplasia
☐ Age at menarche under 14
☐ Age at menopause over 55
☐ Personal history of uterine, ovarian, or colon cancer

_____
Physician's signature

An appointment scheduled for _____ a.m./p.m.

on _____

(Enter referring doctor information here)

Another sample referral form.

PRIVATE CONTRACT FOR MEDICARE PATIENTS

By signing this private contract, the beneficiary or the beneficiary's legal representative:

- Gives up all Medicare coverage of, and payment for, services furnished by _____ _____[doctor and practice name]_____.

- Agrees not to bill Medicare or ask _____[doctor and practice name]_____to bill Medicare for items or services furnished.

- Is liable for all charges of _____[doctor and practice name]_____ without any limits that would otherwise be imposed by Medicare.

- Acknowledges that other supplemental "Medi-gap" insurers may not pay towards the services of _____[doctor and practice name]_____.

- Acknowledges that he or she has the right to receive items or services from other physicians and practitioners for whom Medicare coverage and payment would be available.

- Acknowledges that this is not an emergency or urgent health situation.

_____[doctor and practice name]_____is excluded from participation in the Medicare program under Section 1128 of the Social Security Act.

_____
PATIENT SIGNATURE   DATE

_____
PATIENT'S LEGAL REPRESENTATIVE SIGNATURE   DATE   PHONE NUMBER

_____
PRINT PATIENT NAME

_____
PRINT PATIENT ADDRESS

90

MEDICAL PROBLEMS SUMMARY SHEET

Patient Name:

Medical Problems	Surgeries/Injuries

Health Care Maintenance	Family History
Physical	Mother
Pap	Father
Mammo	ASVD
FOBT	HTN
Sig	DM
PSA	CA
Tetanus	Tobacco
Pneumovax	EtoH
TB	Allergies

A simple summary form for a patient chart.

PARTIAL PROBLEM LIST

Patient Name: _____

Problems: _____

_____

_____

_____

CHP											
Mammo											
BE											
CXR											
ECG/TR											
SIG/COL											
Pap											
CHEM 20											
CBC											
UA											
OB											
GamGlob											
Pneumo					Allergies/Intol						
Hep B											
Tet											
Flu											

Operations/Notes: _____

_____

_____

_____

_____

_____

_____

_____

A summary list is recommended by most professional liability carriers.

PELVIC / PAP EVALUATION

Today's Date: _____

Name _____ Weight: _____ Temp._____ B/P _____

HEENT

CHEST

HEART

BREAST

ABDOMEN

PELVIC   BUSV

CERVIX

UTERUS

ADNEXAL

RECTAL

MENSTRUAL HISTORY

L.M.P. _____

P.M.P. _____

DURATION OF MENSES

SPOTTING/DISCHARGE

MENOPAUSE   ☐ YES   ☐ N0

HYSTERECTOMY   ☐ YES   ☐ NO

OOPHORECTOMY   ☐ YES   ☐ NO

1. GYNECOLOGY—PROBLEMS / SYMPTOMS

2. CURRENT R$_X$ PLAN

A basic annual visit form.

PRESCRIPTION SHEET

Doctor's Lic No. _____ DEA No. _____

Name _____

Address _____

One medication per prescription

Amoxicillin	Tablets	#10	qHS
Augmentin	Chewable	#28	QD
Bactrim	Tablets	#30	BID
Calan SR	Capsules	#50	TID
Diabeta	Solution	#60	QID
Dicloxacillin	Suspension	#100	q AM
Glucotol	Cream	#120	PRN
HCTZ	Ointment	#240	
Hydrocortisone	.1%	100 cc	PO
Ibuprofen	1.0%	150 cc	1 TAB
Insulin 70/30	DS	200 cc	2 TAB
Insulin NPH	.25 mg	15 g	
Insulin Reg	.50 mg	30 g	
Lasix	1 mg	_____	
Lisinopril	5 mg		
Minipress	10 mg		
Multivitamin	20 mg		
Naprosyn	40 mg		
Nystatin	62.5 mg		
Pediazole	125 mg		
Penicillin	250 mg		
Poly vi flor	375 mg		
Propranolol	400 mg		
Tenormin	500 mg		
Tri vi flor	600 mg		
Triamcinolone	800 mg		
Tylenol	_____		

Refill _____ times

☐ No Refill

Signature _____

Doctor's Lic No. _____ DEA No. _____

Name _____

Address _____

One medication per prescription

Amoxicillin	Tablets	#10	qHS
Augmentin	Chewable	#28	QD
Bactrim	Tablets	#30	BID
Calan SR	Capsules	#50	TID
Diabeta	Solution	#60	QID
Dicloxacillin	Suspension	#100	q AM
Glucotol	Cream	#120	PRN
HCTZ	Ointment	#240	
Hydrocortisone	.1%	100 cc	PO
Ibuprofen	1.0%	150 cc	1 TAB
Insulin 70/30	DS	200 cc	2 TAB
Insulin NPH	.25 mg	15 g	
Insulin Reg	.50 mg	30 g	
Lasix	1 mg	_____	
Lisinopril	5 mg		
Minipress	10 mg		
Multivitamin	20 mg		
Naprosyn	40 mg		
Nystatin	62.5 mg		
Pediazole	125 mg		
Penicillin	250 mg		
Poly vi flor	375 mg		
Propranolol	400 mg		
Tenormin	500 mg		
Tri vi flor	600 mg		
Triamcinolone	800 mg		
Tylenol	_____		

Refill _____ times

☐ No Refill

Signature _____

Circle items needed, only one prescription per form, except that additional prescriptions can be written in on the lines provided. Not for use with abusable drugs.

REQUEST FOR RECORDS RELEASE

Physician's Name: _____

Street Address: _____

City: _____ State: _____ ZIP Code: _____

Dear Doctor: _____:

The following individual has asked us to request that his or her medical records be released and forwarded to our office:

Patient Name: _____

Birthdate: _____ Social Security Number: _____

In order for us to fully evaluate this patient's health and make informed decisions, the patient has approved our request for copies of all relevant medical records in your file. Please be sure to include x-ray films and reports.

Thank you for expediting this request. Please send these records to our office address show above.

I hereby authorize the release of all necessary medical records to _____. I wish for them to be forwarded as soon as possible.

Patient's Signature: _____ Date: _____
(or parent if patient is a minor)

Patient's Address: _____ City: _____ State: _____ ZIP Code: _____

Signature of Witness: _____

Call ahead to make sure there will be no charge for copying or to enclose payment to avoid delay.

REQUEST FOR SURGICAL PROCEDURE

Patient Name: _____

Dr. _____ and I have discussed my problem, namely,

_____

Further, we have discussed the procedure for improving this problem,

_____

Alternative means of treatment have been discussed, including

_____

I understand the nature of the procedures as well as the complications

_____

_____

I hereby request, authorize, and give my consent to Dr. _____ to perform upon me the above-named procedures. I further give permission to have anesthetics administered as s/he may deem necessary.

The operation I am to undergo has been explained to me in detail. I understand what is to be done and know that there are certain calculated risks to be taken.
Dr. _____ has not made any guarantee to me whatsoever.

I understand what has been told to me about my condition and what will be done to me.

For aesthetic procedures, I have reviewed and understand the information on the consultation sheet(s) provided to me after my initial consultation with Dr. _____.

_____   _____
Date   Patient Signature

_____   _____
Witness Signature   Doctor Signature

Recommended for any invasive procedure with risks.

102

STAMPS

PROGRESS NOTE STAMP

Date: _____   Temp: _____   Foot Check: _____

Wt: _____   B.P.: _____   L.M.P. _____

Ht.: _____   Pulse: _____   Time in: _____

BLGLU: _____   Resp: _____   Time out: _____

Nursing Orders: _____

RESPIRATORY ILLNESS STAMPS

	NL	
HEAD	☐	_____
EARS	☐	_____
EYES	☐	_____
NOSE	☐	_____
THROAT	☐	_____
NECK	☐	_____
LUNGS	☐	_____
HEART	☐	_____

A stamp for the progress notes for diabetic patients and a stamp for respiratory illness.

SURGERY AND PROCEDURE CONSENT FORM

Date: _____ Time: _____ am/pm

1. I consent to the performance upon _____   _____

(name of patient)   Initials

   the operation or procedure of (technical name): _____

   _____

   The reasons for this operation is (lay language) _____

   and will be performed by _____

and whoever she or he may designate as assistants.

2. The nature and purpose of the operation or procedure, the risks of the operation or procedure.   _____
   and the possibilities of complications have been explained to me, and my questions have been   Initials
   satisfactorily answered.

3. It has been explained to me that a satisfactory result is expected but that the following are some   _____
   of the complications or effects that could or may occur: Initials
   Bleeding, infection, damage to adjacent tissues or organs, swelling, pain, suture reaction,
   delayed healing, scarring, anesthesia or medication reaction, recurrence, additional operations,
   and in rare cases, paralysis or death.

   Additional risks: _____

4. No guarantee has been given by anyone as to the results that may be obtained.   _____

                                                          Initials

5. I consent to the doctors performing whatever different or additional operations or procedures   _____
   they deem necessary or advisable during the course of the operation or procedure.   Initials

6. I consent to the administration of such anesthetics and drugs as may be considered necessary or   _____
   advisable for this operation or procedure except for: _____   Initials

7. I am not known to be allergic and do not have intolerance to anything except: _____
   _____   Initials

8. I understand that I am encouraged and invited to ask any questions I may have, and all of my   _____
   questions have been answered to my satisfaction.   Initials

I HAVE READ AND UNDERSTOOD WHAT THIS FORM CONTAINS.

_____   _____

Patient, parent, or person authorized to sign for patient   Witness to signing

_____

Physician's signature

106

SURGERY LOG

Surgeon: _____   Month: _____

Patient Name	Sched. By	Date Sched.	Surgery Date	ICD-9	CPT	Date Billed	Assisting Surgeon

One way to assure that procedures are organized and billed.

SURGERY SCHEDULING CHECKLIST

pencil only

Patient: _____ Date initiated: _____

Ref. M.D. _____

Surgeon: _____

Proceed ASAP _____ Proceed as soon as practical _____ Proceed see date request _____

Proceed with preauthorization _____ Patient will contact us _____ Other _____

Date Requests _____

_____ Date of procedure as scheduled. (Fill in the other five dates below.)

_____ Time of procedure

<u>AUTHORIZATION</u> (Insurance secretary actually completes this—secretary must notify surgeon if authorized within 48 hours of date initiated. All notes and phone numbers in the process of obtaining authorization are to be kept on the reverse of this page, dated and in chronological order.)

Completed by (initials)

_____ Surgical procedure authorized by _____

_____ Surgical assistant authorized by _____

_____ Hospitalization authorized by _____

<u>BOOKING</u> Date initiated _____

_____ Insurance preauthorization for the operation (hot hospitalization) obtained by

_____ insurance secretary

_____ Second opinion needed? Yes _____ No _____

_____ Arrange second opinion before proceeding with scheduling (use back of this page for notes regarding second opinion) _____, M.D.

_____ Deposit received $ _____ on _____ date by _____

_____ Must be received before scheduling OR date (aesthetic procedures only).

_____ Book: Location _____ Diagnosis _____

_____ Procedures: _____
_____

_____ Date of procedure _____ (1) record date above and fill in other dates in left-hand column and (2) call patient and double-check that patient approves date.

_____ Time _____ Admitting SDS _____ A.M. _____ DBA _____

_____ Anesthesia: Mini _____ Local _____ IV _____ General _____

_____ Schedule anesthesiologist: Yes _____ No _____

_____ Obtain refined cost estimates from hospital regarding operating room and anesthesia costs and record on chart on next page.

_____ Schedule assistant _____, M.D.

_____ Schedule proctor _____, M.D.

_____ Schedule consultant preop _____, M.D.

_____ Special equipment needed: _____

©2003 Professional Management & Marketing

This form provides maximum control and accountability and helps multiple assistants keep track.

SURGERY SCHEDULING CHECKLIST

_____ Autologous blood needed? Yes _____ No_____ No. Units _____

_____ Lab: Applicable for age ____ Platelet _____ PT _____ PTT _____ Bleed time _____

_____ Other test: _____

_____ Schedule second consultation with doctor (15 minutes).

_____ Schedule black and white photographs with doctor (15 minutes).

_____ Schedule preoperative marking (30 minutes): afternoon 1 day prior to surgery
_____, in office day of surgery (2 hours preop) _____
location_____.

_____ Consent signed?

_____ Call admitting (hospitalization expected to be _____ days long).

_____ Place in patient chart: (1) aspirin sheet, (2) laboratory prescription slips, (3) pain
medication Rx, (4) antibiotic Rx, (5) reminder for office to dispense prep solution,
eyeglasses, (6) reminder to be sure patient knows to obtain the necessary garment.

_____ Call patient: (1) date of surgery, (2) date and length of next appointment with doctor,
(3) schedule history and physical, (4) schedule blood donation with center, (5) remind
balance in full to doctor and balance in full by separate check to anesthesiologist due 2
weeks prior to surgery, (6) transportation arranged?

_____ DATE: TWO AND A HALF WEEKS PRIOR TO SURGERY

_____
_____ Call patient: (1) history and physical scheduled? (2) confirm need for payment in full,
separate check for remaining balance for doctor and separate check for entire balance
for anesthesiologist, (3) confirm next appointment, (4) inform patient of refined cost
estimates for hospital/anesthesia fees.

_____ DATE: TWO WEEKS PRIOR TO SURGERY

_____ Patient comes to office for second consultation and brings final payment.

_____ *Has written insurance authorization arrived? Yes ____ No ____ N/A _____

_____ How is this authorization requirement fulfilled? _____

_____ Check if second opinion is necessary? Is it completed? Yes _____ No _____

_____ *Full payment received by doctor? Date _____

_____ *Full payment received by anesthesiologist? Date _____

_____ Sent to anesthesiologist _____

_____ Patient makes payment to hospital cashier. Date _____

_____ Check—black and white photographs taken? Yes _____ No _____

_____ When scheduled? _____

_____ Check—call physician to perform history and physical examination. Confirm
appointment and date arranged and ask for copy to be sent to doctor.

_____ Patient received: (1) aspiring sheet, (2) pain medication Rx, (3) antibiotic Rx, (4) prep
solution, (5) glasses, (6) other _____

_____ Patient knows about garment to be obtained? Yes _____ No _____

_____ Arrangements now complete _____

_____ Autologous blood donation completed? Yes _____ In progress ____ No _____

_____ When arrangements were/are to be completed _____

_____ Arrange dried flowers at OR for patient pickup after surgery (aesthetic surgery only).

©2003 Professional Management & Marketing

SURGERY SCHEDULING CHECKLIST

_____ DATE: WEEK PRIOR TO SURGERY

_____ Black and white film taken to photographer?

_____ Pick up black and white prints from photographer and have for doctor as soon as possible for preoperative evaluation.

_____ Check if doctor is to be H&P. Is it dictated? Yes _____ No _____

_____ Reminder given to doctor.

_____ Call patient: ask—(1) any snags in obtaining H&P, (2) pain med Rx, (3) antibiotic Rx, (4) prep solution, (5) garment, (6) blood donation

_____ *Remind patient not to take any aspirin or aspirin-containing products

_____ Remind patient to bring garment to preoperative marking session so it can be doubled-checked.

_____ DATE: DAY OF SURGERY

_____ Write date of surgery in office chart notes and name of procedure.

_____ Copy of (1) initial consultation, (2) office notes, (3) operative permit, (4) booking sheet photocopied and on doctor's desk to take to surgery the next day.

_____ Obtain phone number where patient will be the evening postoperatively. Put this phone number on the doctor's index card next to patient name and date of surgery.

_____ *Check—is there enough time scheduled for doctor to complete examination of last scheduled office patient, drive to OR, and still be in the OR 15 minutes before the scheduled procedure? Is there also scheduled additional time for preoperative markings and history and physical as needed?

_____ Call the OR, request special equipment noted on previous page. (If no special equipment is noted, ask doctor if there are any special requirements.)

** Congratulations! You successfully completed all these arrangements again!

Quotes	Estimate	Refined Estimate	Actual
Surgical			
OR Fee			
Anesthetic Fee			
H&P/Lab/X-ray fee			

DATE: ONE MONTH AFTER SURGERY

_____ Obtain actual costs from patient for (1) operating room fees, (2) laboratory fees,

_____ (3) history and physical fee, (4) anesthetic fee and record in chart above.

** Cancellation OR **Date/Time Change:
1. Remove previous date and time from schedule
2. Call patient
3. Call OR desk
4. Call assistant surgeon
5. Call proctor
6. Change all dates of this form (above)

114

X-RAY AND IMAGING APPOINTMENT REQUEST

X-RAY AND IMAGING APPOINTMENT REQUEST

Patient Name: _____

Date of Exam: _____ Time: _____

Referring M.D, _____ Phone: _____

Area of Interest:

☐   MRI   _____

☐   CT Scan   _____

☐   Ultrasound   _____

☐   Mammogram   _____

☐   Fluoroscopy   _____

☐   General X-ray   _____

☐   Other   _____

☐   Old Films   Date _____ Place _____

Scheduled appointments are preferable for MRI, CT, Ultrasound, and Fluoroscopy.

Lab work may be done at the time of the exam.

Indication for exam: _____

_____

_____

_____

Maybe you can get your imaging center to provide referral slips to you. Consider a check box of locations on a generic form if you use different centers.

REFUSAL OF TREATMENT BY PATIENT

REFUSAL OF TREATMENT BY PATIENT

Patient _____ Age _____

Date _____ Time _____ Place _____

I have been advised by Doctor _____ that it is recommended

for me to undergo the following treatment, operation or procedure: _____

_____

_____

The risks, benefits, and alternatives of this treatment have been explained to me.

Although my failure to follow the advice I have received my seriously impair my health or life, I nevertheless refuse the recommended treatment, operation, or procedure.

Specific risks of refusing my doctor's recommendation include:

_____

_____

_____

I assume the risks and consequences involved and release Dr. _____ from any liability.

Signed: _____ Date: _____

Witness: _____ Date: _____

118

SPECIALTY REFERRAL AUTHORIZATION

Authorization No. _____

(Date of Expiration)

SPECIALTY REFERRAL AUTHORIZATION

Health Plan: _____

❏ Commercial
❏ Medicare HMO
❏ Medicaid

_____
PATIENT'S Name

_____
Street Address   City   State   Zip   Telephone #

                                                                      M   F
_____
Identification Number   Patient Hospital (Pool)   Date of Birth   Sex

PCP _____ PCP Phone # _____ Per Patient Request?   YES   NO

TO BE COMPLETED BY PRIMARY CARE PHYSICIAN'S OFFICE

MEDICAL JUSTIFICATION FOR REFERRAL _____   YES   NO
                        Date of PCP Visit   Diagnosis (ICD9 code)   Report Attached?

History & PE/Prior Workup/Prior Treatment _____
_____
_____
_____

Retroactive approval of emergency referral? YES   NO   If YES, date referral made _____   Other _____

SPECIALIST SERVICES REQUESTED _____
                        CPT(s)   Service/Procedure   Type of Specialty

ICD9(s) _____ Description _____   # of Visits Requested

SPECIALIST requested   Street   City   State   Zip   Phone Number

Location/Hospital   Street   City   State   Sip   Phone Number

PCP SIGNATURE _____

TO BE COMPLETED BY SPECIALTY PHYSICIAN'S OFFICE

SPECIALTY PHYSICIAN REPORT _____   YES   NO
                        Date of Visit   Diagnosis (ICD9 code)   Report Attached?
Findings and Recommendations _____
_____
_____
_____

Recommended Treatment Plan for PCP _____
_____
_____

Specific Procedures Requested _____
_____

❏ IN Patient ❏ OUT Patient ❏ In OFFICE Date(s) of Service _____ Number of Visits: 1 2 3 4 5 6

SPECIALIST SIGNATURE _____

TO BE COMPLETED BY MEDICAL GROUP

❏ APPROVED   ❏ NOT APPROVED   Date _____

MEDICAL DIRECTOR (or designee) SIGNATURE _____

(AUTHORIZATION IS SUBJECT TO MEMBER ELIGIBILITY AND PLAN BENEFITS)

GENERIC REFERRAL SLIP

Date:

Dear:

I am referring _____ for evaluation in your office.

This patient's diagnosis is:

I am referring this patient for evaluation of:

Pertinent history or physical examination findings include:

Pertinent Labs or X-rays:

Other significant information:

Your evaluation of this patient is greatly appreciated. If you have any further questions, please do not hesitate to call me.

Sincerely,

122

ENT REFERRAL SLIP

ENT REFERRAL   Appointment Date:

Date:

Dear:

I am referring _____ Birthdate _____

for evaluation of:

      Recurrent tonsillitis _____

      Recurrent otitis media _____

      Chronic sinusitis _____

      Other _____

Pertinent history:

      Treatment of this condition began on _____

      Episodes of otitis media _____

      Number of episodes of tonsillitis _____

      Number of episodes of culture positive strep _____

      Significant snoring and/or obstructive breathing _____

      Antibiotics utilized thus far include: _____

      _____

      Other significant history or physical findings: _____

      _____

Your evaluation, as always, is greatly appreciated. Please call me if you have any further questions.

Sincerely,

SPECIALIST EVALUATION AND RESPONSE TO REFERRAL

TO: _____, M.D.

FROM: _____

Today's Date: _____

Re: PATIENT NAME _____

Patient Date of Birth _____

Date of Pt. Visit at: _____

Insurance: _____

I.D. # _____

Thank you for referring the above identified patient to _____. This mutual patient was seen on the above date for_____
Our findings were _____
_____

Copies of any/all results from tests ordered will be sent to your office.

We recommend this patient be seen at _____ for _____
on _____ and are therefore requesting a referral/authorization from you.
At your earliest convenience, please fax this form back to us with the referring physician. Please feel free to contact our office at _____ should you require further information.

Thank you for your assistance.

....

For referring physician office to use in authorizing the above patient visit to Dr. _____

☐ Appointment with physician is authorized based on the above information.
    M.D. authorizing visit for pt. (please print M.D. name) _____
    M.D. signature: _____ Date: _____

☐ Appointment not authorized: Reason: _____
_____
    By: _____

☐ Please call referring physician office at (ph. #): _____
    and speak with _____

Please fax this completed page back at your earliest convenience to _____

Thank you.

TEST RESULTS NOTICE TO PATIENT

_____

_____

_____

Date: _____

Regarding your: Blood Test _____   Pap Smear _____
                 Cholesterol _____   Urinalysis _____
                 Mammogram _____   X-Ray _____
                 Other _____

☐ All results within normal limits

☐ With the exception of _____

_____

☐ Please make an appointment for a follow up visit in:

        _____ Days
        _____ Weeks
        _____ Months

☐ This test should be repeated in _____

Comments: _____

_____

_____

_____

CONSULTATION AND REFERRAL REQUEST

Date: _____

Patient: _____

Referring Physician: _____

Referred to: _____

Tentative Diagnosis: _____

Priority:
☐ Emergency
☐ 72 Hours
☐ Routine

Requested Involvement:
☐ Evaluate and return patient with recommendations for management.
☐ Evaluate and treat for this particular problem, then return patient.
☐ Assume management of patient within your field of expertise.

If Surgery or Special Procedure is Indicated:
☐ Please notify referring physician as he wishes to participate.
☐ Please proceed without participation of referring physician.

History:

Positive Physical Findings:

Lab and X-ray Findings:

Medication or Procedures Already Utilized:

Other Information:
☐ Pertinent lab and x-ray reports are enclosed.
☐ The patient will hand carry pertinent lab data or x-rays for your review.
☐ Pertinent lab or x-rays pending at the time of this referral

_____
Signed

GYNECOLOGICAL RECORD

Name: Age: Date:

CC:

PI:

LMP: PMP:

OMP: (pads/day) IMB: PCB:

Leukorrhea Monilia Trichomonas

VD:

Dysmenorrhea Dyspareunia

Intercourse Frequency Orgasm

Papanicolaou smear: Result:

Hormones:

Medications:

Parity: Full term Premature Abortion Living

	Year	Labor	Weight	Result	Location and Complications
1					
2					
3					
4					

Surgeries & Hospitalizations:

Accidents:

Blood Transfusions:

X-ray Rx:

Allergic Reactions:

Husband: Age Diabetes TB Leukemia

Twins

Family: F M S B

Diabetes TB Leukemia

CNS Diseases Twins CA

Social: Born Raised Educated: HS

College

Grad

Travel:

Habits: Smoking   Pack/day   for   years   Alcohol
                                                                         Coffee
                                                                         Tea

ROS:

    Head:
    Eyes:
    Ears:
    Nose:
    Throat: Dental:
    Neck: Thyroid:
    CR:
    GI: Appetite   Maximal: BM
                           Present Weight: Acholia
                                  Minimal: Yellow Jaundice
                                                        Melena
                                                Hematochezia
                                              Hemorrhoids

    GU: Infections
                    Dysuria   Pyuria   Hematuria   Calcauria
                    Frequency   Hesitancy   Urgency   Retention
                    Urinates   x/day   x/night   Stress Incontinence

    NM: Joints   Muscles

OSTEOPOROSIS PREVENTION ASSESSMENT SUMMARY

Name: _____   Social Security #: _____

Address: _____   Phone: _____

_____   Birth Date: _____

Type of Medical Insurance: Primary _____ Secondary: _____
(Please present your insurance cards at the time of visit so we can copy them)

1. Ethnic background: _____
2. Is there a family history of: Loss of height with age? _____
   Dowager's hump? _____
   Hip fracture? _____

3. Do you have a history of: Surgery? _____   Type: _____
   _____
   Prolonged bed rest? _____
   Broken boned? _____ Which bones? _____
   Back pain? _____
   Arthritis? _____

4. Have you had any radionuclide or radiopaque substances in your body in the past week? _____
5. Age at last menstrual period: _____ Number of pregnancies: _____
6. Is there a possibility that you may be pregnant? _____

7. Medications   (Present)   (Past)

   _____   _____

   _____   _____

   _____   _____

   _____   _____

Do you:
8. Regularly drink milk or eat dairy products? (Present)_____ (Past) _____
   If yes, how many ounces daily? (1 cup = 8 oz.) (Present) _____ (Past) _____
9. Regularly take a vitamin or mineral supplement? _____
   If yes, indicate the name of supplement and how often you take it. _____
   Drink five or more cups of coffee or soft drinks daily? _____
10. Have more than 2 ounces of alcohol daily? _____
11. Smoke? _____ Past or Present? _____ How many years? _____
12. Exercise? _____ What type? _____ How often? _____
13. Referring Physician (if any) _____

14. Date: _____

* *

Our assistant will measure your height and weight at the time of your visit.

Ht: _____ Wt._____ Arm span: _____

IMAGING REQUEST

Date: _____

Patient Name: _____

Patient Date of Birth: _____

Patient Age: _____

Motion or communication special needs: _____

Insurance Plan/ID # _____

Referred by name: _____

Referred by phone: _____

X-ray   ☐

Mammogram   ☐

CT   ☐

MRI   ☐

Ultrasound   ☐

Fluoroscopy   ☐

Other   ☐   _____

Anatomical site(s) _____

_____

_____

_____

Clinical indications/diagnosis: _____

_____

_____

_____

SPECIALIST REFERRAL LIST

Specialty: _____

Dr/Clinic Name: _____

Phone #: _____

Fax #: _____

Pager #: _____

E-mail: _____

Diagnosis or Tx preference: _____

Plans accepted: _____

Specialty: _____

Dr/Clinic Name: _____

Phone #: _____

Fax #: _____

Pager #: _____

E-mail: _____

Diagnosis or Tx preference: _____

Plans accepted: _____

Specialty: _____

Dr/Clinic Name: _____

Phone #: _____

Fax #: _____

Pager #: _____

E-mail: _____

Diagnosis or Tx preference: _____

Plans accepted: _____

LAB RESULTS

CONTACT TRACKING LOG

Today's Date	Patient	Test	Normal Result Y N	Contacted by	Notes

142

OPHTHALMOLOGY LENS DISPENSARY QUESTIONNAIRE

Help us determine your eyewear needs by filling out the following eyecare lifestyle assessment form. Your answers will assist us in formulating a personalized and complete presentation of your eyewear options.

1) Does your work require you to focus at a variety of distances? _____
2) Are you satisfied with the visible lines in your current bifocals? _____
3) Would you be interested in a product which could improve night vision? _____
4) Are you troubled by glare and ghost images created by your lenses? _____
5) Would you be interested in a lens that could unmask your eyes because it is virtually "invisible"? _____
6) Does the weight of your current lenses make your glasses uncomfortable? _____
7) Do you work around power equipment? Are you involved in active sports? Is eye safety a concern of yours? _____
8) Would you be interested in learning more about lenses which are specially designed to answer the demands of: Driving? _____ Boating? _____ Skiing? _____ Shooting? _____ Tennis? _____ Check the appropriate line. Other? _____
9) You probably already protect your skin from the sun's harmful burning rays, but did you know that a single afternoon of unshielded exposure to the sun could temporarily diminish your eyes capacity for night vision by as much as 90%? Would you like to learn more about ultraviolet eye protection? _____
10) Do you operate a computer? _____ Does your computer screen cause you to have eyestrain? _____ Do you ever have neck or back stiffness, and/or headaches often associated with computer posture problems? _____
11) Would you like to protect your investment in plastic lenses and insure longer wear by adding an extra measure of scratch protection to the surface of your lenses? _____
12) Does road surface, snow, or water glare create a problem for you? Would you be interested in learning more about the only lens which effectively eliminates glare? _____
13) Would you be interested in learning more about lenses that automatically adjust to any lighting condition? _____
14) Does the thickness of your current lenses concern you? Would you like to learn more about new lends materials and special edge treatments that could serve to reduce thickness and add cosmetic appeal to your lenses? _____
15) In general, are you interested in learning more about the latest and best products that the optical industry has to offer? _____

In addition to the general areas already outlined, do you have any specific occupational and/or recreational endeavors which may require additional "visual" attention? Briefly list your comments below.

_____
_____
_____
_____

Thank you for taking the time to help us better serve your needs.

POST PARTUM GYN EXAM

INTERNAL USE ONLY

Name _____ Age _____ Date _____
Wt _____ Ht _____ BP _____ UA _____ Hb _____
Pregnancy Weight _____ Weight before delivery _____
Concerns _____
_____

S:LNMP _____ Flow (lt) (med) (heavy) Clots _____ Duration _____ Cramps _____
Pain/blood with intercourse _____ Regular _____ Frequency q. _____
G _____ P _____ AB _____ TAB _____ Last Pap _____ (NI) (Abn) _____
SBE YES NO Itching? _____ Abnl vg D/C _____ Breast Lumps YES NO
Date of Delivery _____ Vaginal/C/Section _____ Reason for C/Section _____
Complications _____ When did bleeding stop? _____
Sexually active yet? _____ Contra before IUP _____ Contra now _____
Support at home? YES NO Breast feeding? YES NO Any problems? _____

PM Hx
_____
_____

Δ's PM Hx
_____
_____

Habits
Smoke_____
ETOH _____
Caffeine _____

FM Hx
_____
_____

Δ's FM Hx
_____
_____

Exercise
What _____
Duration _____
Frequency _____

Medications
_____

Allergies
_____
_____

Diet
Low fat _____
5 veg/fruit/day _____
Dairy _____
Grains _____
Red meat/wk _____

General Apprnce _____	Breasts _____
Skin	
Thyroid	
Heart	
Lungs	
Abd	Cervix
Ext Gen	
Vault	
Uterus ANT ML RETRO	
Adnexa (R) (L)	Rectal

A/P
  #1 HCM pap _____
  mammo _____
  SBE _____
  _____
Δ's Diet _____
Δ's Habits _____
Δ's Exercise _____

#2 _____
_____
_____
#3 _____
_____
_____
_____

SPECIAL SEXUAL FUNCTION

Date: _____

Your responses to the items on this questionnaire will allow us to make a preliminary decision about arrangements necessary for the proper diagnostic and treatment program.

1. IDENTIFICATION INFORMATION
Name _____
Address _____
           Street   City   State   Zip
Occupation _____
Birth Date _____
Present Marital Status   S   M   W   D
No. Previous Marriages _____
Your Doctor's Name _____
Your Doctor's Address _____
Your Doctor's Phone Number _____ Area Code _____
Your Doctor's Specialty _____ General Practice _____
   Urology _____ Other (Specify) _____
Would you like us to send copies of our findings to your physician? _____ Yes _____ No

2. Please describe in your own words your past sexual history; include in this description your current problem and how this problem affects your life. (If more space is needed, use back of page.)
_____
_____
_____

3. Please give a brief description of your social-educational background (parent, marital status, children, social environment, etc.); include the items that you feel may be important to us in assessing the potential value of this treatment or in selecting the best treatment to suit your case.
_____
_____
_____

4. CHARACTERISTICS OF ERECTION
a) Do you have erections at all? _____ Yes _____ No
b) Are you able to get sufficient erection to make vaginal penetration? _____ Never _____ Rarely _____ Half the time _____ Most of the time _____ Always
c) Do you ever awaken in the morning with an erection? _____ Yes _____ No
   If so, is it _____ full, _____ partial, or _____ poor?
d) Have you noticed a change in the firmness of these early morning erections? _____ Yes _____ No
e) Does the quality of your erections improve occasionally? _____ Yes _____ No
f) Do you notice any curvature of the penis during erection? _____ Yes _____ No
g) Did the start of your current erection problem happen _____ suddenly _____ slowly _____ currently happening intermittently
h) Did you experience an extremely stressful event around the time your erection problem began? ____ Yes ____ No
i) Do you find it easier to obtain an erection while on vacation? _____ Yes _____ No

5. CHARACTERISTICS OF PENIS
   Are you concerned about the size of your penis? _____ Yes _____ No
   If so, what is the problem? _____

6. CHARACTERISTICS OF ORGASM OR CLIMAX
a) Do you now have orgasms or climaxes? _____ Yes _____ No
   If so, how often? _____
   If not, how often before your problem developed? _____
   If so, how is orgasm achieved? _____
      vaginal penetration _____
      by hand _____
      orally _____
      conventional method with partner but without penetration _____
      other (describe) _____
   If so, does semen (sperm) or liquid come out? _____ Yes _____ No

148

b)   Can you masturbate to climax?   _____ Yes _____ No
     If so, does the penis get hard then?   _____ Yes _____ No
c)   Do you experience "premature" ejaculation?   _____ Yes _____ No
d)   Do you experience pain with ejaculation or climax?   _____ Yes _____ No

7.   CHARACTERISTICS OF SEXUAL DESIRE
a)   How strong is your desire for sexual intercourse? _____ Poor _____ Fair _____ Strong _____ Very Strong
b)   How strong is the desire of your wife or sexual partner? _____ Poor _____ Fair _____ Strong _____ Very Strong
c)   How long with current sexual partner? _____
d)   What is your partner's attitude about your having an operation to treat impotence? _____

8.   PAST MEDICAL HISTORY
a)   Have you seen a doctor for treatment of your problem?   _____ Yes _____ No
     If so, please describe the treatment and results: _____
b)   Have you consulted any kind of mental health counselor (specialist, psychiatrist, psychologist, or social worker)
     about your problem?   _____ Yes _____ No
     If so, describe when and the results (include name and address) _____
c)   Do you take any daily or weekly medications?   _____ Yes _____ No
     If so, list them and indicate purpose: Drug: _____ Dosage: _____ Purpose: _____
d)   How often do you drink alcoholic beverages?
     1.   Never
     2.   Once or twice a year
     3.   Once or twice a month
     4.   Every weekend
     5.   Several times a week
     6.   Every day
e)   How much do you drink?
     1.   don't drink
     2.   1 drink
     3.   2-3 drinks
     4.   4-7 drinks
     5.   8 or more drinks
     6.   until "high" or drunk
f)   What is your usual drink? _____
g)   Do you use any "street drugs"?   _____ Yes _____ No
     If so, please name _____
h)   Do you use tobacco products?   _____ Yes _____ No
     If so, how much? _____
i)   Have you had surgery in the past?   _____ Yes _____ No
     If so, please list: Surgery _____ Date _____ ____
j)   Have you had any serious accidents?   _____ Yes _____ No
k)   Do you have any history of the following:
     Heart disease _____
     High blood pressure _____
     High cholesterol _____
     Pain in legs, thigh or hips with walking or exercising _____
     Numbness in your penis or legs _____
     Diabetes _____
     Headaches _____
     Prostatitis or urinary tract infections _____
     Thyroid disorders _____
     Difficulty sleeping _____
     Appetite change _____
     Change in bowel habits _____
     Difficulty with urination _____

9.   Is there any further information you feel is important to your problem? _____
     _____

RESPIRATORY MEDICAL HISTORY

Name _____

Social Security No. _____

Date _____

Company/Department _____

Sex _____ Date of Birth _____ Age _____

Questionnaire administered by _____

I. Occupational history: Please list entire work history starting with present job and going back to first job. (Use extra sheet if necessary.)

Industry (or company) and location	From	To	Specific job

	Yes	No	Number of years
A. Have you ever worked in a dusty job?			
1. In a mine?			
2. In a quarry?			
3. In a foundry?			
4. In a pottery?			
5. In a cotton, flax, or hemp mill?			
6. With asbestos?			
7. In a brick plant?			
8. As a sandblaster?			
9. In the manufacture of glass, ceramics, or abrasives?			
10. In other dusty jobs? Specify _____			

	Yes	No	Number of years
B. Have you ever worked with chemicals?			
1. Solvents? Specify _____			
2. Acids? Specify _____			
3. Lead?			
4. Plastics? Specify _____			
5. TDI?			

152

	Yes	No

II.   Previous illnesses

    A.   Have you ever been told you have any of the following problems?

        1.   Asthma?

        2.   Emphysema?

        3.   Chronic bronchitis?

        4.   Pneumonia?

        5.   Tuberculosis?

        6.   Pleurisy?

        7.   Heart trouble of any type?

III.   Symptoms

    A.   Cough

        1.   Do you usually cough first thing in the morning?

        2.   Do you usually cough at other times during the day or night?

Skip 3 to 6 if answer to 1 and 2 is "no." Answer if "yes."

        3.   Do you cough on most days for as much as 3 months of the year?

        4.   For how many years have you had this cough?

           Less than 2 years _____

           2 to 5 years _____

           5 years or more _____

        5.   Do you cough more on any particular day of the week?

           If yes, which day? _____

        6.   Do you cough during any particular season of the year?

           If yes, which season?_____

    B.   Sputum

        1.   Do you usually bring up phlegm, sputum, or mucus from your chest first thing in the morning?

        2.   Do you usually bring up phlegm, sputum, or mucus from your chest at other times of the day or night?

Skip 3 and 4 if answer to 1 and 2 is "no." Answer if "yes."

        3.   Do you bring up phlegm, sputum, or mucus from your chest on most days for as much as 3 months of the year?

        4.   For how many years have you raised phlegm, sputum or mucus from your chest?

           Less than 2 years _____

           2 to 5 years? _____

           5 years or more? _____

    C.   Wheezing

        1.   Does your breathing ever sound wheezy?

        2.   Have you ever had attacks of shortness of breath with wheezing?

        3.   Have you ever had a feeling of tightness in your chest?

Skip 4 to 6 if answer to 1, 2, or 3 is "no." Answer if "yes."

        4.   At what age did wheezing first occur? _____

        5.   How frequently does wheezing occur?

           Daily _____

           Nightly _____

           A few times per week _____

           A few times per month _____

           A few times per year _____

        6.   Is it worse on any particular day of the week?

           Which day? _____

©2003 Professional Management & Marketing

154

		Yes	No

D. Breathlessness
   1. Do you get short of breath when walking on level ground?
   2. Do you get short of breath while walking up stairs?
   3. How many flights of stairs can you climb up without stopping?
      1 to 2? _____
      2 to 3? _____
      More than 3? _____
E. Hemoptysis
   1. Have you ever coughed up blood from your chest?
      If yes, when was the last time this happened? _____			

IV. A. Smoking (presently) 1. Do you now smoke regularly (cigarettes, pipe, cigars)?			
Skip 2 to 6 if answer to 1 is "no." Answer if "yes."	2. How old were you when you started smoking? _____ 3. For how many years have you smoked regularly? _____ 4. How many cigarettes do you now smoke each day? _____ 5. How much pipe tobacco do you now smoke each week? _____ 6. How many cigars do you now smoke each day? _____		
B. Smoking (formerly) 1. Have you ever smoked regularly?			
Skip 2 to 7 if answer to 1 is "no." Answer if "yes."	2. How old were you when you started smoking regularly? _____ 3. For how many years did you smoke regularly? _____ 4. How long ago did you last quit smoking? _____ Months _____ Years _____ 5. How many cigarettes did you usually smoke per day? _____ 6. How much pipe tobacco did you usually smoke per week? _____ 7. How many cigars did you usually smoke per day? _____		

V.   Additional comments

156

BRIEF DERMATOLOGY HISTORY

Welcome to our office! In order to give you the best, most comprehensive care possible, please provide us with the following information. All information is confidential and released only with your written permission.

Your Name (please print): _____

Today's Date: _____

Please explain your skin concerns/questions: _____
_____

If you have a skin problem, when did you first notice it? _____

Where is it? _____

Please circle "YES" or "NO" and answer the following; make any comments in the space provided below the questions.

Have you had any other skin problems? If yes, please list.   Yes   No
_____

Does anyone in your family have skin problems or skin cancers?   Yes   No
_____

Are you now being treated by a doctor?   Yes   No

Dr. Name _____ City _____ For What? _____

Has a doctor given you anything for your skin? If yes, please explain below.   Yes   No
What? _____

Have you put anything else on your skin yourself? If yes, please explain below.   Yes   No

_____

Are you allergic to any medications? (Penicillin, Aspiring, etc.) Please list.   Yes   No
_____

Does anything touching your skin cause a rash or allergy? Please list below.   Yes   No
_____

Please list all pills, medicines, vitamins, etc. that you are taking. (Both prescription and over-the-counter). _____
_____

Is there anything else I should know about your health? (such a recent surgery, diabetes, high blood sugar, ulcers, easy bleeding, etc.). If yes, please explain.   Yes   No
_____
_____

Are you pregnant?...Yes   No

Are you taking hormones or birth control pills? ....Yes   No

Have you ever been treated by a dermatologist before?....................................Yes   No

For skin problems?...Yes   No

For cosmetic reasons..Yes   No

Please identify: ❑ collagen   ❑ vein treatment   ❑ surgical procedures   ❑ mole removal   ❑ hair loss

158

CONSENT TO OPERATION AND OTHER MEDICAL SERVICES/PROCEDURES

Date _____ Time _____

1. I authorize the performance upon _____ of the
    (patient's name)

    following operation _____

    to be performed under the direction of Dr. _____

2. The following have been explained to me by Dr. _____ :

    A. The nature of the operation _____
        (description of operation)

        _____

    B. The purpose of the operation _____

        _____

    C. The possible alternative methods of treatment _____

        _____

    D. The possible consequences of the operation _____

        _____

    E. The risks involved _____

        _____

    F. The possibility of complications _____

        _____

3. I have been advised of the nature of the operation and have been advised that if I desire a
    further and more detailed explanation of any of the foregoing or further information about
    the possible risks or complications of the above listed operation, it will be given to me.

4. I do not request a further and more detailed listing and explanation of any of the items listed
    in paragraph 2.

Signed _____ **Date** _____

Witness _____

160

BRIEF PRE-SURGERY QUESTIONNAIRE

In an effort to serve you better, we request that you provide us with the following information. We need this information to give you the best care and treatment possible. All information is held strictly confidential and is only released with your written consent.

Last Name:	First:	Age:	Sex:

Doctor's Notes
Please do not write in this area

Presenting Problem or Proposed Surgery:

ILLNESS/INJURY: Please check if you have ever had:

Yes	No		Yes	No	
		High blood Pressure			Abdominal bleeding
		Diabetes			Diverticulosis
		Peptic Ulcers			Thyroid problem
		Heart Attack			Lung problems/Asthma
		Chest pain/tightness			Shortness of breath
		History of heart murmur			Accidents/Broken Bones: (please list)
		Stroke			
		Cancer			
		Hepatitis			
		Yellow Jaundice			
		Gallstones			
		Kidney Stones			

OPERATIONS: Please list names and dates of all operations you have had: ☐ none

Year	Name of Operation	Type of Anesthetic if known	Complications

Have you ever had a blood transfusion? ☐ No ☐ Yes Date: _____

List any hospital admissions or medical conditions not listed above: _____
_____

Females only – Are you pregnant? ☐ No ☐ Yes

DRUGS Please list all drugs you are taking and their dosage:			**ALLERGIES** Type of reaction & name of medication	
Drug Dosage	Drug	Dosage	Name of Drug	Reaction

Do you smoke or have you smoked?	# of Cigarettes_____	☐ Per Day ☐ Per Week	# of Years_____ Quit _____
Do you drink alcohol? Quit? _____	Type _____	Ounces _____	☐ Per Day ☐ Per Week

The above information is true and accurate.

Patient Signature (or parent if patient is a minor) _____ Date _____

INFORMED CONSENT FOR EXERCISE TESTING

INFORMED CONSENT FOR EXERCISE TESTING

In order to determine an appropriate plan of medical management, I hereby consent to engage voluntarily in an exercise test. The information thus obtained will determine the state of my heart and circulation, as well as the activities I may engage in safely.

The test will be performed on a treadmill, the speed and grade of which will be increased gradually. This increase may continue until symptoms such as fatigue, shortness of breath, or chest discomfort appear, until adequate heart rate is achieved, or until significant abnormalities on the heart monitor are identified.

Historically treadmill testing has been safe; however, possible risks include an abnormal blood pressure response, an irregular heart beat (too rapid, too slow, or ineffective), fainting and very rarely heart attack or death. Every effort will be made to minimize the risk by preliminary examination, and by careful observation during testing. Specialized equipment and trained personnel are available both on site and within close proximity to deal with unusual situations should they arise.

I have read and understand the foregoing. Any questions which may have occurred to me have been answered to my satisfaction.

_____
Patient Signature   Date

_____
Physician Supervising Test   Date

_____
Witness Signature   Date

PATIENT STERILIZATION AUTHORIZATION

PATIENT STERILIZATION AUTHORIZATION

Date and time _____

We, the undersigned husband and wife, each being more than twenty-one years of age and of sound mind, authorize _____, M.D. and assistants of his choice to perform the following operation, bilateral partial vasectomy, upon _____.
      (patient)

It has been explained to us that this operation is intended to result in sterility although this result has not been guaranteed. We understand that a sterile person is NOT capable of becoming a parent.

Signed _____ (husband)

Signed _____ (wife)

Signature Witnessed:

By _____

By _____

TELEPHONE TRIAGE GRID SAMPLE

Type of Call	Stat to ER	Stat to Dr.	To Dr.	To RN	Take Msg	Other
Fever over _____						
Fever under _____						
Choking						
Bleeding wound						
Menses problem						
Overdose						
Physician personal						
Physician referring patient						
Record request						
Insurance Co. calls						
CPA or attorney call						
Family calls						

CHICKEN POX (VARICELLA) VACCINE

WHAT IS CHICKEN POX?

Chicken pox is a common viral illness. Although it can create a lot of discomfort, it is usually not dangerous or life threatening. This involves a rash made up of tiny blisters, which can last up to 10 days and may be very itchy. Chills, headache, and a loss of appetite may also occur.

WHAT HARM CAN IT DO?

Complications resulting from chicken pox rarely can be skin infections, pneumonia or encephalitis (brain infection). These can be serious enough to require hospitalization in some, and extremely rarely might cause death. Most of these very serious complications occur in adults with chicken pox. Once someone has had chicken pox, this virus stays forever silently in the person. Later in life, the virus can reappear as shingles which can cause pain and blisters.

WHO IS AT RISK FOR GETTING CHICKEN POX?

Chicken pox most commonly occurs between 6 and 10 years of age. However, some people will not get chicken pox until they are teens or adults, when it is more severe and lasts longer than childhood chicken pox. Those with impaired immune function are especially susceptible.

WHAT IS CHICKEN POX VACCINE?

This is a vaccine against the chicken pox disease, similar to other vaccines such as measles or polio. It causes the body to produce immunities to protect against the disease and gives a person 70 to 90% protection. Children less than age 13 should be vaccinated with a single dose. Children older than 13 would receive two doses of the vaccine four to eight weeks apart.

WHY SHOULD YOU CONSIDER THE VACCINE FOR YOURSELF OR YOUR CHILD?

The vaccine should be considered as an alternative to prevent the complications of chicken pox mentioned above. Most groups recommend the vaccine for children 11 years and older who have never had the chicken pox, adults who have not had chicken pox and who are at high risk for exposure (such as child care and health care workers), and any children or adults who live with a family member with a weakened immune system (such as leukemia, HIV, or organ transplant patient). However, the American Academy of Pediatrics recommends the vaccine for all children between 12 and 18 months who have not already had chicken pox. They also recommend older children be immunized at the earliest opportunity. This last recommendation at present is a bit controversial because there may not be enough supply of vaccine to meet that expectation. Because vaccinated people will not get chicken pox, they will also be protected from getting shingles in the future.

WHAT ARE THE SIDE EFFECTS OF THE VACCINE?

Reactions to the vaccine are generally mild and might include the following: Redness, stiffness, soreness, and swelling around the area where the shot is given; a rash of small bumps or pimples around the site of the shot; fatigue (feeling very tired); fever; nausea; fussiness in infants and young children.

WHO SHOULD NOT RECEIVE THE VACCINE?

The following people should **not** receive the vaccine: pregnant women; breast feeding women; anyone with a disease or medical treatment which suppresses the immune system.

WARNING

There is a chance that after completing the immunization, a person could still get chicken pox. If you experience any reaction, report it at once to your doctor. If you have any further questions about this, ask your doctor.

CONSENT

I have read and understand the contents of this form, including the potential risks of the vaccine, even the risk of failure to protect against chicken pox. I understand no guarantee can be made to me regarding these issues, and I've had my questions answered.

I decided **to receive** the vaccine   I decided **not to receive** the vaccine.

_____   _____
Signed   Relationship   Signed   Relationship

Date: _____   Date: _____

*Financial Forms*_____

Introduction

The business office is where most of the paperwork really occurs. Computers often generate great mountains of information in a format that is not easily digestible. Many of the forms in this section are geared toward analysis and reporting formats that help with management of the data. Other business office forms are in the Managed Care and Insurance sections.

We purposely left out some of the most common forms, such as CMS-1500s, 10- and 15-minute increment schedule book pages, superbills, and others, because they are either standard, extremely customized or widely available.

ACCOUNTS RECEIVABLE AGING REPORT

Month:_____

Date Performed: _____
Performed by: _____

Payer	0-30	31-60	61-90	90+	Notes
Patient Portion					
Medicaid					
Medicare					
Worker's Comp					

Use for management review periodically.

ACCOUNTS RECEIVABLE MANAGEMENT BONUS WORKSHEET

Collection Ratio

Determine the historical collection ratio for the practice.　　　　_____
Determine specialty comparable collection ratio.　　　　　　　_____
Determine the target collection for the practice.　　　　　　　_____

Bonus staff $X for each month they beat the target ratio.　　　_____

AR Aging

Determine the historical AR aging.　　　　　　　　　　　　_____
Determine specialty comparable AR aging.　　　　　　　　　_____
Determine the target AR aging.　　　　　　　　　　　　　_____

Bonus staff $X for beating target or Y% of difference between target and actual total AR below target.

　　　　　　　Example:　　$100,000 AR target
　　　　　　　　　　　　$90,000 actual AR with 1% of difference bonus
　　　　　　　　　　　　$10,000 difference x 1% = $100 bonus paid

or

Bonus staff similar to above but for AR over X days (60 or 90)　　_____

or

Bonus staff X% of all collections　　　　　　　　　　　　　_____

176

BUSINESS SUMMARY

20___

Mo	# Days Wrkd	Charges	Collections	Adj	Accounts Receivable	Tot New Pts	Tot Vists	Avg Vists/Day	Hosp Pts.	Hosp Charges	Overhead		Notes
Jan													
Feb													
Mar													
Apr													
May													
Jun													
Jul													
Aug													
Sep													
Oct													
Nov													
Dec													
Total													

A useful form for spotting trends. Should be provided to doctor monthly.

CHARGES/RECEIPTS—ANNUAL COMPARISON

Charges	200__	200__
Jan		
Feb		
Mar		
Apr		
May		
Jun		
Jul		
Aug		
Sep		
Oct		
Nov		
Dec		
TOTALS		

Receipts	200__	200__
Jan		
Feb		
Mar		
Apr		
May		
Jun		
Jul		
Aug		
Sep		
Oct		
Nov		
Dec		
TOTALS		

Accounts Receivable   Total _____   _____ $_____
                                       month   year

Accounts Receivable Aging   0–30 _____   31-60 _____

                                 61-90 _____   90+ _____

Do monthly or quarterly if more detailed forms are not used.

CHECKLIST FOR PRACTICE BILLING SYSTEM AUDIT

Date: _____ By: _____

	Yes	No
• Current CPT code book or minibook—does it look used?	☐	☐
• ICD-9-CM book volumes 1 and 2 (diagnostic reference)	☐	☐
• Current HCPC listing for each state the practice bills	☐	☐
• Binder of Medicare, Medicaid, BCBS, indemnity, HMO newsletters, correspondence	☐	☐
• File of HMO/PPO/IPA contracts	☐	☐
• Charge sheets (office, hospital, nursing home)	☐	☐
• Service and revenue report	☐	☐
• Fees adjusted in last six months	☐	☐
• Reimbursement records by payer	☐	☐
• Process of reviewing rejections and down coding, quantity • reasons • repetition • reporting	☐	☐
• Are modifiers being used adequately?	☐	☐

A periodic audit is a good idea, especially after a staff change. If the doctor or manager or CPA is not able to do the audit, call in a consultant.

COLLECTION AGENCY ACCOUNT TRACKING

Agency name _____

Contact person _____   Phone _____

Patient Name	Date Sent	Date Paid	Amount

COLLECTION LETTER 1 (SOFT)

Dear Patient:

It is the policy of this office to contact patients who have received two billing statements but have not replied. We are certainly aware of the difficult financial times in which we are now living, and because of this we think communication between our office and patients regarding past-due bills is most important.

We ask that you cooperate in calling our office to communicate with us about your outstanding balance. We are certain we can work out a suitable written payment arrangement with due dates, amounts, etc., to the benefit of all. Keep in mind that we accept VISA/MasterCard for payment in full on accounts.

We thank you for your cooperation and look forward to assisting you.

Sincerely,

Bookkeeper

COLLECTION LETTER 1 (HARD)

Re:

Dear:

An audit of your account indicates an overdue balance of $ _____.

If this is correct, please pay it immediately by cash, check, or credit card.

If it is incorrect, please call our office at _____.

This balance may consist of a previous unpaid fee, copayment after insurance, or insurance payment denied or uncollectible from your insurance company. Payments unpaid by your insurance company are your responsibility.

IF THIS ACCOUNT IS NOT PAID, CORRECTED, OR PAYMENT ARRANGEMENTS MADE BY _____, IT WILL BE SENT TO A COLLECTION AGENCY.

You may incur additional costs and be reported to a national credit reporting agency.

We certainly hope you give this matter your immediate attention.

Sincerely,

Bookkeeper

COLLECTION LETTER 2

To:

From:

Date:

Re: Payment Arrangements

This is to verify our telephone conversation of _____.

We agreed that you will be paying $_____ by the _____ of each month to complete payment of your professional fees. The total balance owing is $_____. You will be paying _____ payments, with the final payment being made on the _____ of _____.

Please sign below for our records and return one copy of this letter to our office in the enclosed envelope. We have also enclosed a copy for you to keep for your records. We appreciate the opportunity to provide you with the medical care you need.

Approved:

_____   _____
Patient Date   Date

_____   _____
Office Representative   Date

COLLECTION LETTER 3

To:

Date:
Balance Due:

Final Notice

Because your account is long past due, we would normally turn it over to a collection agency. We would, however, prefer dealing directly with you since a collection agency action would affect your overall credit rating. Please read and check one of the options below and return this signed form to us by _____.

_____   1.   I would prefer to settle this account. Please find full payment enclosed.

_____   2.   I would prefer to make monthly payments. Please see attached for my payment commitment.

_____   3.   I prefer to have this balance paid in full by my:
                          VISA/MasterCard (circle one)
                          Exact name on account: _____ Exp. date _____
                          Total amount authorized _____

_____   4.   I would prefer that you send my account to collections or move to legal action.

OFFICE USE ONLY: Voucher prep'd. _____   Verif no. _____

Date verif _____   Copy to chart _____   Copy to pt _____

IF FULL PAYMENT OR REGULAR PAYMENTS ARE NOT MADE, FURTHER ACTION WILL BE TAKEN BY _____.

If you have any questions, call the office at _____.

192

COLLECTION LETTER 4

Date:

Name:

Address:

Our records show that you have not responded to our ☐ letter ☐ conversation ☐ telephone conversation regarding your check no. _____, dated _____. That check was made payable to our business and was returned to us by your bank.

We are prepared to proceed to court action unless payment in full on the amount below is received by _____.

Amount of check	$ _____
Bank service charge	$ _____
Total due now	$ _____

Any person who writes a bad check or any order for payment of money which is dishonored for lack of funds may be civilly liable and may be sued for damages plus the amount of the check and court costs.

Our court action against you will be in the amount of $_____ plus court costs.

You should be aware that these damages are allowed by law in a CIVIL action such as small claims and do not take the place of any criminal prosecution that may be imposed by local law enforcement officials.

Sincerely,

Bookkeeper

CREDIT CARD ACCEPTANCE

We now offer "Charging by Mail"!

You can now make payments on your account using your VISA, MasterCard, or American Express card. If you want to take advantage of this new service, please complete the bottom half of this form and return it to us along with the top portion of your statement in the provided envelope.

Thank you!

Yes, I would like to make a payment of $ _____.

Please charge my   □ VISA   □ MasterCard   □ American Express

Card Number: _____ MasterCard No.: _____
                                                             (found above your name)

Authorized Signature: _____ Exp. Date _____
                            (required)

Print name: _____ Address: _____

City: _____ State: _____ ZIP: _____

VISA, through your bank, may also offer a "signature on file" plan for patients that is valid for one year. It is useful for primary care practices and those with repetitive appointments.

Provider/Dr. Name _____

E & M CODING WORKSHEET

Patient Name: _____   Time in: _____

☐   Outpatient or Office……………..   ☐ New (3 Key) or ………... ☐ Established (2 of 3 Key)

☐   Hospital…………………………   ☐ Initial (3 Key) or ………. ☐ Subsequent (2 of 3 Key)

☐   Consultations, Office (3 Key)

☐   Consultations, Inpatient…………   ☐ Initial (3 Key) …………. ☐ Follow-up (2 of 3 Key)

☐   Confirmatory Consultations {2nd or 3rd opinions} (3 Key)

☐   Emergency Department (3 Key)

☐   Nursing Facility………………..   ☐ Initial ……………….....☐ Annual

    …………………………………..   ☐ Admission (All 3 Key) ….☐ Subsequent (2 of 3 Key)

☐   Domiciliary, Rest Home,

☐   Custodial Care………………..   ☐ New (3 Key) …………….☐ Established (3 Key)

☐   Home Visit…………………..   ☐ New (3 Key) …………….☐ Established (3 Key)

History	Exam	Number of Diagnosis or Management Options	Amount and/or Complexity of Data to Be Reviewed	Risks of Complications and/or Morbidity or Mortality	DECISION MAKING (2 OF 3)
[ ] Problem Focused	[ ] Problem Focused	[ ] Minimal	[ ] Minimal or none	[ ] Minimal	[ ] Straightforward
[ ] Expanded Problem Focused	[ ] Expanded Problem Focused	[ ] Limited	[ ] Limited	[ ] Low	[ ] Low Complexity
[ ] Detailed	[ ] Detailed	[ ] Multiple	[ ] Moderate	[ ] Multiple	[ ] Moderate Complexity
[ ] Comprehensive	[ ] Comprehensive	[ ] Extensive	[ ] Extensive	[ ] Extensive	[ ] High Complexity

☐ Over 50% of visit time spent counseling
Ancillary Services Provided:

Time Out: _____

Procedure Codes(s): _____

For doctors who still refuse to code their own evaluation and management visits and have the staff to do it.

EQUIPMENT COST ANALYSIS
WILL THE WIDGET SAVE ENOUGH TIME?

To calculate if an instrument will "pay for itself in
time saved," use the following formula.

	Formula		
	Purchase price ÷ estimated useful life in years	=	
+	Annual cost of supplies and maintenance	+	_____
=	New instrument's annual cost	=	_____
÷	Days/times used per year	÷	_____
=	**Cost per day/time used**	=	

Staff Labor:

	Wage per hour		
+	Benefits per hour	+	_____
=	Labor cost per hour	=	_____
÷	60 (minutes per hour)	÷	_____
=	**Staff labor cost per minute**	=	

Doctor Labor:

	Annual receipts		
÷	Hours worked per year	÷	_____
=	Gross receipts per hour	=	_____
÷	60 (minutes per hour)	÷	_____
=	**Doctor labor cost per minute**	=	

Time Savings Needed: Doctor   or   Staff

	Cost per day
÷	Labor cost per minute
=	**Minimum no. of minutes needed**
	to be saved per day/times used to justify cost

To calculate additional profit potential

	Reimbursement for service
-	Reimbursement w/o new equipment
=	Increased reimbursement per procedure
-	Additional labor per procedure
-	Other (remodel, training, space used)
-	Cost per time used (above)
=	Profit per procedure
X	Estimated procedures per year
=	**Profit per year**

Remember: In addition to time saved, the widget may also increase reimbursement, add services, or just be too much fun to pass up.

EXPENSE-SHARING GROUP ACCOUNTING REPORT

for the month of _____ 20___

Expenses
Divided by Productivity

Physician Extended Wages	$ _____			
Physician Extended Benefits	$ _____			
Staff Wages	$ _____			
Clinical Supplies	$ _____			
Office Supplies	$ _____			
Repairs	$ _____			
_____	$ _____	Dr. A _____%	Dr. B _____%	Dr. C _____%
Subtotal	$ _____	$ _____	$ _____	$ _____

Divided Equally 3 Ways

Legal and Accounting	$ _____			
Outside Services	$ _____			
Marketing	$ _____			
_____	$ _____	Dr. A 1/3	Dr. B 1/3	Dr. C 1/3
Subtotal	$ _____	$ _____	$ _____	$ _____

Divided Equally 4 ways (C=2)

Janitorial/Maintenance	$ _____			
Rent and Utilities	$ _____			
Telephone	$ _____			
Business Insurance	$ _____			
Waiting Room Magazines	$ _____			
_____	$ _____	Dr. A ¼	Dr. B ¼	Dr. C ½
Subtotal	$ _____	$ _____	$ _____	$ _____

Other/Miscellaneous

_____	$ _____	$ _____	$ _____	$ _____
_____	$ _____	$ _____	$ _____	$ _____
Subtotal	$ _____	$ _____	$ _____	$ _____

Expenses per Physician Total	$ _____	$ _____	$ _____	$ _____
Expenses Paid by Tenants	$ _____	$ _____	$ _____	$ _____
_____	$ _____	$ _____	$ _____	$ _____
_____	$ _____	$ _____	$ _____	$ _____

FEE EXPLANATION

Dear Patient:

Your fee for service includes your visit with the doctor based on the time and complexity of your condition and any treatment provided. In addition, proper attention to your case requires that the doctor spend more time working for you outside your direct visit with him or her. such time may include:

- Creation of a permanent medical record.
- Review of all laboratory blood test results (e.g., a biochemical survey and CBC contain 42 separate test to interpret and file in your chart).
- Review of prior and current x-ray or scan reports and personal review with the radiologist of abnormal studies.
- Preparation and mailing of consultation reports and follow-up visits letters and laboratory/scan results to referring physicians and any subsequent consulting.
- Follow-up phone call or letter regarding laboratory test results of patients and/or copies of test results when indicated or requested.
- Phone consultation with referring or consulting physicians and other health care providers about your case.
- Other phone calls to and from you and your family members for various reasons.
- Referral letters to any further specialists recommended by the doctor.
- Patient educational materials and medication samples when available.
- Any research done by the doctor about your case. The doctor used medical libraries and computerized medical search services.
- Staff assistance regarding your visit.
- Arranging and coordinating other tests and consultations.
- Calls to and from pharmacies.
- Insurance application forms: health insurance, disability insurance, life insurance.
- Insurance reports: health claims, disability claims to insurance and state, Medicare disability.
- Discussions (sometimes acrimonious) with hospitalization utilization review, insurance companies, or Medicare for ongoing hospitalization.
- Review and management of hospital records.
- Letters of necessity to obtain medical instruments or prescriptions.
- Letters of necessity for medical services to insurance companies.
- Arrangements for hospitalization with hospital admissions, house staff physicians and consulting physicians, and test/treating facilities.
- Communication daily during admission with nurses, house staff, and attending physicians.
- Tumor registry and other required reports.
- Home health care and nursing facility orders.
- Other reports and forms: jury duty, school, job, sick leave, back to work, communicable disease, etc.

In addition, the doctor participates extensively in continuing medical education, clinical research, teaching, and medical writing to keep up-to-date on the latest medical advances.

At our office, we feel a strong commitment to keep costs to our patients down. Even so, the cost of salaries, rent, taxes, insurance, billing, postage, photocopying, medical supplies, office supplies, medical journals and textbooks, and other materials keeps increasing. We charge only what we feel is necessary in order to maintain the highest standard of care. We look forward to a lasting and healthy relationship with you.

Sincerely,

A very good form to give to any patient who is surprised by or upset at the bill. We do not recommend giving it to all patients without need.

SCHEDULE OF PAYMENTS

Pmt No.	Due Date	Amount of Installment	Date Paid	Follow Up
1				
2				
3				
4				
5				
6				
7				
8				
9				
10				
11				
12				
13				
14				
15				
16				
17				
18				
19				
20				
21				
22				
23				
24				
25				
26				

FINANCIAL AGREEMENT

For professional services rendered.
Patient, or parent of patient if patient is a minor:

1. Cash professional fee for services $ _____
2. Cash down payment (incl. deductible) $ _____
3. Estimated insurance payment $ _____
4. Uninsured balance $ _____
5. Amount financed $ _____
   (the amount of credit provided to you)
6. Finance charges $ _____
   (the dollar amount the credit will cost you)
7. Annual percentage rate $ _____
8. Total of payments $ _____
9. Total of amount $ _____
   (1 + 6 above; sum of cash amount, financing
   charge, and any amounts financed by creditor)

Total payments (8 above) is payable to Dr. _____ in _____ monthly installments of $ _____ each and _____ installments of $ _____ each. The first installment is due on _____, and following installments on the same day of each consecutive month until paid in full.

NOTICE TO PATIENT/GUARDIAN

Do not sign this agreement if it contains any blank spaces. You are entitled to an exact copy of any agreement you sign. You have the right at any time to pay the unpaid balance due under this penalty without penalty. You have a right at this time to receive an itemization of the amount financed.

☐ I want an itemization   ☐ I do not want an itemization

I have read, understood, and agreed to the above financial agreement, terms and conditions, and schedule of payments.

_____   _____
Signature of responsible party   Date

_____   _____
Doctor's signature   Date

A variation of the federal truth-in-lending form used when interest is charged, a finance fee is charged, or an extended payment plan is offered. We recommend not charging interest or a finance fee and using that policy as a marketing tool to the patient. Always check the itemization box and provide a copy of the superbill or billing summary. Give the patient a copy.

INCOME AND EXPENSES STATEMENT—BASIC

Period: _____   Total Receipts: _____

Income	Amount	% of Total Receipts
Ancillary Provider Wages		
Ancillary Provider Benefits		
Staff Wages		
Staff Benefits		
Legal and Accounting		
Outside Services		
Janitorial/Maintenance		
Rent and Utilities		
Clinical Supplies		
Office Supplies		
Telephone/Ans. Service/Pager		
Malpractice Insurance		
Business Insurance		
Dues		
Journals		
Continuing Education		
Marketing		
Entertainment		
Taxes		
Repairs		
Lab Fees		
Postage		
Loan Payments		
Miscellaneous		
Replacement Reserve/Depreciation		
Subtotal		

Owner/Doctor Wages: _____   _____

Owner/Doctor Benefits: _____   _____

Auto Expense: _____   _____

Life/Disability Insurance: _____   _____

Total: _____   _____

Profit: _____   _____

Decide with your CPA. Use a CPA who has many physician clients.

STATEMENT OF INCOME AND EXPENSES - CASH BASIS - DATE_____

QUARTER			YEAR TO DATE	
CURRENT YR/%	PRIOR YR/%		CURRENT YR/%	PRIOR YR/%

		Charges		
		Adjustments		
		NET CHARGES		
		Collections		
		Refunds		
		NET COLLECTIONS		
		Staff Wages		
		Staff Benefits		
		Staff Retirement Plan		
		Staff Continuing Education		
		Outside Services		
		Janitorial/Maintenance		
		Donations and Contributions		
		Dues		
		Furniture/Equipment		
		Insurance - Business/Other		
		Insurance - Malpractice		
		Interest on Loans/Credit Cards		
		Journals & Books		
		Laboratory/Radiology		
		Lease payments - Equipment		
		Legal, Accnting & Consultants		
		Marketing - Ads/Meals/Ent		
		Meals - Business/Staff Mtgs		
		Miscellaneous		
		Postage/FedEx/Courier		
		Rent and Utilities		
		Repairs & Maint - Building		
		Repairs & Maint - Equipment		
		Retirement Plan-Fees		
		Supplies - Clinical		
		Supplies - Administrative		
		Taxes & Licenses		
		Telephone/Ans Service/Pager		
		Travel and Prof Meetings		
		Uniforms and Laundry		
		OPERATIONAL EXPENSE SUBTOTAL		
		EMPLOYED PROFESSIONALS:		
		Doctor Assoc Wages		
		Doctor Assoc Benefits		
		Doctor Assoc Retirement Plan		
		Doctor Assoc Continuing Ed		
		Ancillary Wages (PA/FNP/PT)		
		Ancillary Benefits		
		Ancillary Retirement Plan		
		Ancillary Continuing Ed		
		ANCILLARY COSTS SUBTOTAL		
		DOCTOR-OWNER:		
		Salary/Wages/Draw		
		Auto		
		Continuing Ed/Dues/Journals		
		Marketing - Ent		
		Insurances/Life/Health		
		Other		
		Retirement Plan		
		COMPANY NET INCOME (LOSS)		

209 ©2003 Professional Management & Marketing

Decide with your CPA. Use a CPA who has many physician clients.

INTERNAL AND MISCELLANEOUS FINANCIAL CONTROLS
(target dates and guidelines)

- Balancing out the accounts receivable (either by computer or manually by adding up ledger cards to cross-check with day sheets) will take place monthly by the _____.
- Patients with outstanding balances will have bills sent out to them by the _____ of each month.
- All billings to patients will have "all bills due and payable in full by the _____ of the month."
- Billings to patients in which insurance has been billed and we are awaiting payment will have a stamp, message, or sticker noting this.
- Aging reports will be completed monthly. Breakdowns will include 30, 60, 90, and 120+ categories and will also be broken down by major type of category (M/Care, M/cal, HPR, privates, etc.). Accounts will be aged by computer by the _____ of each month.
- A comprehensive review of accounts receivable will be performed monthly with doctor and office manager between the _____ and the _____ of each calendar month. (Generally takes place at the monthly management meeting.)
- Routine follow-up accounts receivable/collections or insurance follow-up will take place monthly between the _____ and _____ of each month.
- Superbills will be numbered, and a numerical tracking system will therefore exist. Superbills with errors, etc., will be kept for tracking and accountability.
- Write-offs of over _____% will be reviewed with the doctor monthly. This is for monitoring, coding, strategy, and general assessment of carriers and payment levels.
- Insurance billing will be completed/up to date for the practice at least _____

  _____

  Should billing or processing of claims get behind the above schedule, office manager will report it promptly to doctor. The plan for solution will include a written proposal and time line for bringing processing up to date. (This issue is particularly important as you document the need to expand staffing. All changes in staffing/additions to staffing will be supported by the real need in this way.)
- Deposits will be made at least _____ times per week and/or made daily if more than $_____ in receipts exists.
- The bank statement for the practice will be on a calendar month closing.
- The bank statement will be mailed to the doctor's house and reviewed. The statement will be brought into the office by the doctor within _____working days of receiving it.
- The business checking account will be balanced monthly by the office manager by the _____ of each month. Documentation of balancing will be kept and a report made at the management meeting monthly regarding results.
- All incoming bills will be stamped with the date received into the office and placed immediately into the accounts payable 1 through 31 tracking file for payment.
- Payables will stay in the folder/file until paid. Problem or question bills will be placed on the doctor's desk within _____ working days of receipt for disposition and returned back to the office manager within _____ working days for action.
- All payables will be mailed out a minimum of _____ days prior to the date they are due. Bills will be paid on the _____ and the _____ of each month.
- Checks written will be accompanied by the stub, payment coupon, or some type of documentation for doctor review when signing the check. No check will be approved by doctor without some type of verification. A copy of the verification will be maintained with the payment date, amount, and check number on the paperwork.
- Closeout on general ledger will take place monthly with the last entry on the last day of each month.
- Balancing (totals) on the payables/general ledger will be completed by the _____ of each month.
- A running balance will be kept in the check register at all times.
- Spreading the information in the general ledger will take place as the check is posted.
- A petty cash journal will be kept and balanced monthly. A fund of $ _____ will be kept (locked). When the fund gets below $25, the officer manager will replenish it.
- When paying cash, a patient will receive a receipt with notation on the account.

212

INTERNAL FINANCIAL CONTROL CHECKLIST

By: _____ Date: _____

	Yes	No
Cash Collections and Receipts		
Is a change fund being maintained?	☐	☐
Are receipts issued for cash payments	☐	☐
Are receipts prenumbered?	☐	☐
Are carbon copies of receipts kept?	☐	☐
Are payments received indicated as check or cash on the receipts and daysheets/computer?	☐	☐
Is cash totaled daily to agree with daysheets/computer?	☐	☐
If a receipt is spoiled, is it voided and left in the book attached to daysheet?	☐	☐
Are employees who handle cash bonded?	☐	☐
Deposits		
Is deposit prepared daily?	☐	☐
Are deposits held overnight stored safely?	☐	☐
Are the carbon copy deposit slips attached to the daysheet/computer run?	☐	☐
Is the bank statement opened only by the doctor or accountant?	☐	☐
Is the bank statement mailed to the doctor's home?	☐	☐
Does amount deposited to business account from receipts balance with month-end totals?	☐	☐
Daysheets and Financial Cards		
If on a manual/pegboard system, is it used correctly?	☐	☐
Is there an individual daysheet/computer run for each day?	☐	☐
Does the doctor review and initial the daysheets/computer run?	☐	☐
Are daysheets/daily computer runs compared with appointment book and financial records monthly?	☐	☐
If manual:		
-Are daysheets and financial cards prepared in ink?	☐	☐
-Is a tape of accounts receivable cards run at the end of each month and balanced with A/R on daysheets?	☐	☐
-Are financial cards stored safely?	☐	☐
-Are all financial cards returned to card files nightly?	☐	☐
Are all accounts with balances billed?　Even those pending insurance?	☐	☐
If computerized, where possible, are billing and collection duties done by separate persons?	☐	☐
Is backup on the computer performed daily?	☐	☐
Are disks stored off site in a safe place?	☐	☐
Petty Cash		
Do you itemize cash expenditures?	☐	☐
Are receipts kept for petty cash expenditures?	☐	☐
Do you keep a running balance of petty cash?	☐	☐
Does the cash balance agree with the records? Is it balanced monthly?	☐	☐
Are employees' purses and personal belongings kept in a separate location away from front office area?	☐	☐
Employees		
Are employees required to rotate duties and responsibilities where possible?	☐	☐
Are refund checks approved by the doctor?	☐	☐
Are "write-offs" and adjustments reviewed by the doctor monthly?	☐	☐
Are accounts in internal collection contacted at least monthly?	☐	☐
Accounts Payable and Miscellaneous		
Does doctor sign all checks?	☐	☐
Do you refuse to keep a signature stamp in the office?	☐	☐
Does the doctor refrain from "skimming" or "dipping" into the petty cash?	☐	☐
Do you have your CPA or an outside person perform periodic reviews?	☐	☐

(We recommend monthly internal cross checks; this takes only about 20 minutes a month.)

This form allows you to audit financial controls and discourage embezzlement.

OB FINANCIAL AGREEMENT EXPLANATION SHEET

Welcome and congratulations as an OB patient

INSURANCES Our office will check with your carrier to see if OB care is included with your coverage. Your insurance will pay: _____

GENERAL INFORMATION

Your full OB professional fee will be $ _____.
This amount covers your initial exam, routine/normal prenatal care, and the physician delivery charge for a **normal vaginal delivery**. Complicated vaginal delivery or cesarean delivery will add additional professional fees since it requires specialized care.

Some additional laboratory charges will be incurred due to testing required during pregnancy monitoring. These lab and handling charges are not included and will be billed to you separately. Injections will also be billed to you separately and are not included in the above amount. Some optional testing may be recommended.

Hospital charges, anesthesiology, medications, extra hospital supplies, or any items provided by the hospital will be billed to you directly from the hospital and are not included in our fee as stated herein.

A six-week follow-up postdelivery visit with the doctor will be required **and is included** in your OB fee. There will be lab testing required in coordination with this postdelivery visit. These charges will be billed to you separately.

A thorough check of your baby in the hospital will be completed and will be chargeable separately.

Payment schedule: Patient Name: _____ Projected Due Date: _____

	Date due	Payment Amount	Balance due
1)	_____	_____	_____
2)	_____	_____	_____
3)	_____	_____	_____
4)	_____	_____	_____

There will be no late charge and no interest chargeable on your account.

We comply with all consumer protection truth-in-lending guidelines for payments. All fees for prenatal care and delivery are due and payable in full before the projected delivery date. Our office policy requires payment in full of the patient portion for all OB care by the eighth month of pregnancy. This financial agreement is to be agreed to and signed by both patient and office manager and explains what is covered and what is not.

Dr. _____ is in a call/coverage group. Every effort will be made to be available for your delivery; however, occasionally it will be necessary to call upon one of these physicians in our community.

Thank you for selecting us for your OB care. It is the highest compliment we can receive.

I have read and understand this agreement and agree to abide by its terms.

_____   _____
Patient Signature and Date   Office Manager Signature and Date

FINANCIAL POLICY

Patient Name: _____ Date of Birth: _____

BASIC POLICY Pay for service is due in full at the time service is provided in our office.

FOR PATIENTS WITH INSURANCE We bill most insurance carriers for you if proper paperwork is provided to us. We will also bill most secondary insurance companies for you. Copayments and deductibles are due at the time of service. Since your agreement with your insurance carrier is a private one, we do not routinely research why an insurance carrier has not paid or why it paid less than anticipated for care. If an insurance carrier has not paid within 60 days of billing, professional fees are due and payable in full from you.

MEDICARE PATIENTS We will bill Medicare for you. We will also bill secondary insurance carriers for you. All copayments or deductibles are due and payable at the time service is provided.

WELFARE PATIENTS All welfare patients must provide a current, valid sticker before being seen.

SURGERY FEES All copays, deductibles, and payments for noncovered surgical procedures are due prior to your surgery. Prior authorization may be required by your carrier.

NONCOVERED SERVICES Any care not paid for by your existing insurance coverage will require payment in full at the time services are provided or upon notice of insurance claim denial.

PERSONAL INJURY CASES This office does not bill for auto accident or other liability or lawsuit-related cases. You are responsible for payment at the time of service. We do not accept liens.

WORKER'S COMPENSATION If your injury is work-related, we will need the case number and carrier name prior to your visits in order to bill the worker's compensation insurance company.

YEARLY HEALTH CHECKS Periodic preventive health checks may or may not be covered under your health insurance policy; however, they may be required by your physician.

MISSED APPOINTMENTS In fairness to other patients and the doctor, we required at least 24 hours' notice to cancel appointments. You may be charged for missed appointments or dismissed from the practice.

OB FINANCIAL GUIDELINES These are covered in our OB fact sheet.

Please check on: I have paid my insurance deductible for the calendar year _____ ☐ Yes ☐ No ☐ Don't know

MEDICARE PATIENTS: SIGNATURE ON FILE I request payment of authorized Medicare benefits be made either to me or on my behalf to _____ for any services furnished me by the listed provider/supplier. I authorize any holder of medical information about me to release to the Health Care Financing Administration and its agents any information needed to determine these benefits or the benefits payable to related services.

I understand my signature requests that payment be made and authorizes release of medical information necessary to pay the claim. If "other health insurance" is indicated in Item 9 of the CMS-1500 form or elsewhere on other approved claim forms or electronically submitted claims, my signature authorizes releasing of the information to the insurer or agency show. In Medicare assigned cases, the provider or supplier agrees to accept the charge determination of the Medicare carrier as the full charge, and the patient is responsible only for the deductible, coinsurance, and noncovered services. Coinsurance and the deductible are based upon the charge determination of the Medicare carrier.

Patient's Name (Please Print):	**PROVIDER**
Patient's Signature:	
Patient's Medicare No.: Date:	

ASSIGNMENT OF INSURANCE BENEFITS Patients with insurances please read and sign below.
I hereby assign all medical and/or surgical benefits, to include major medical benefits to which I am entitled, private insurance, and any other health plans, to _____. This assignment will remain in effect until revoked by me in writing. A photocopy of this assignment is to be considered as valid as an original. I understand I am financially responsible for all charges whether or not paid by said insurance. I hereby authorize said assignee to release all information necessary to secure the payment.

Signature: _____ Date: _____

I have read, understood, and agreed to the above financial policy for payment of professional fees.
The patient is ultimately responsible for all professional fees.

Signature: _____ Date: _____

PATIENT ENCOUNTER FORM

Patient Name: _____ Date: _____

Insurance: _____ Prev Balance: _____

NEW PATIENT			Fee
Visit Expanded	☐	99202	_____
Visit Detailed	☐	99203	_____
Visit Comp.	☐	99204	_____
Visit Consult.	☐	99205	_____

Well Child

Infant (<-1 yr)	☐	99381	_____
Child (1-4 yr)	☐	99382	_____
Child (5-11 yr)	☐	99383	_____
Child (12-17 yr)	☐	99384	_____

Annual Exam

18-39 years	☐	99385	_____
40-60 years	☐	99386	_____
65 years and over	☐	99387	_____

ESTABLISHED PATIENT

Nurse Visit	☐	99211	_____
Visit Focused	☐	99212	_____
Visit Expanded	☐	99213	_____
Visit Detailed	☐	99214	_____
Visit Comp.	☐	99215	_____

Well Child

Infant (<-1 yr)	☐	99391	_____
Child (1-4 yr)	☐	99392	_____
Child (5-11 yr)	☐	99393	_____
Child (12-17 yr)	☐	99394	_____

Annual Exam

18-39 years	☐	99395	_____
40-60 years	☐	99396	_____
65 years and over	☐	99397	_____
OB Package	☐	59400	_____
Annual GYN	☐	90089	_____

INJECTIONS			Fee
Allergy.	☐	95120	_____
Hepatitis B	☐	90723	_____
DTP	☐	90701	_____
DT	☐	90702	_____
Flu Vac.	☐	90659	_____
Gamma Glob.	☐	90393	_____
HIB	☐	90647	_____
MMR	☐	90707	_____
Pneumo Vac	☐	90732	_____
Rubella	☐	90706	_____
Tine	☐	86585	_____
Versed	☐	90782	_____
Lidocaine	☐	90782	_____

PROCEDURE

Anoscopy	☐	46600	_____
Audiometry	☐	92551	_____
Avul/Nail	☐	11730	_____
Burn tx	☐	16000	_____
Casting	☐	29___	_____
Colonoscopy	☐	45378	_____
w/Biopsy	☐	45380	_____
Colposcopy	☐	57452	_____
w/Biopsy	☐	57454	_____
Cyro/Cervix	☐	57511	_____
Cyro/Skin	☐	17340	_____
I&D Abscess	☐	10060	_____
Inj. Trig. Pt.	☐	20550	_____
Inj. Inter. Jt.	☐	20605	_____
Inj. Major Jr.	☐	20610	_____
Pap	☐	88147	_____
(w/handling fee)	☐	99000	_____
Tonometry	☐	92100	_____
Tympanometry	☐	92567	_____

PROCEDURE cont			Fee
Vasectomy	☐	55250	_____
Surgery	☐	_____	_____
Other	☐	_____	_____
Other	☐	_____	_____

LABORATORY

Blood Sugar	☐	82948	_____
Chlamydia	☐	87490	_____
Hematocrit	☐	85014	_____
Hemoccult	☐	82270	_____
Monospot	☐	86308	_____
Pap	☐	88150	_____
Preg UA	☐	81025	_____
Strep Screen	☐	87880	_____
UA Complete	☐	81000	_____
UA Chem	☐	81005	_____
UA Culture	☐	87088	_____
Wet Mount	☐	87210	_____
Pap (handling fee)	☐	99000	_____
Other	☐	_____	_____
Other	☐	_____	_____

SERVICES

Record Pap	☐	99080	_____
Other	☐	_____	_____

SUPPLIES

Sterile Tray	☐	99070	_____
Orthopedic	☐	_____	_____
Other	☐	_____	_____
Other	☐	_____	_____

DIAGNOSIS

☐ Abscess 682.9
☐ Abdominal Pain 789.0
☐ Acne 706.1
☐ Adjustment Dis 309.28
☐ Allergies 995.3
☐ Amenorrhea 626.0
☐ Anemia 285.9
☐ Annual Gyn Exam V70.0
☐ Annual PE V70.1
☐ Anxiety 300.0
☐ Arrhythmia 427.9
☐ Arthritis 716.9
☐ ASHD 414.0
☐ Asthma 493.9
☐ Backache 724.5
☐ Breast Mass 611.72
☐ Bronchitis 490
☐ Bursitis 727.3
☐ CAD 414.0
☐ Cervical Dysplasia 622.1
☐ Chest Pain 786.5
☐ CHF 428.0
☐ Conjunctivitis 372.30
☐ COPD 496
☐ Contraception V25.09

☐ Cough 786.2
☐ CVA 436
☐ Depression 311
☐ Dermatitis 692.9
☐ Diabetes 250.0
☐ Duodenal Ulcer 532.9
☐ Dysmenorrhea 625.3
☐ Ear Impaction 380.4
☐ Fatigue 780.7
☐ Fever 780.6
☐ Fracture _____
☐ Gastritis 535.05
☐ Gastroenteritis 558.9
☐ Gout 274.9
☐ Headache 784.0
☐ Hematuria 599.7
☐ Hemorrhoids 455.6
☐ HIV Human Immunodeficiency Virus 042
☐ Hypertension 401.9
☐ Hyperlipidemia 272.4
☐ Hypothyroidism 244. 9
☐ Irritable Bowel 564.1
☐ Low Back Pain 724.2
☐ Lymphadenopathy 785.6
☐ Menopausal Syndrome 627.2
☐ Mono 075

☐ Nausea/Vomiting 787.02
☐ Obesity 278.0
☐ Osteoporosis 733.00
☐ Pancreatitis 577.0
☐ PID 614.9
☐ Pharnygitis 462
☐ Pneumonia 486
☐ Pregnancy V22.2
☐ Rectal Bleeding 569.3
☐ Scabies 133.0
☐ Sinusitis 473.9
☐ Soft Tissue Injury _____
☐ STD _____
☐ Substance Abuse _____
☐ Tendonitis 726.90
☐ Tinnitis 388.30
☐ UTI 599.0
☐ URI 465.9
☐ Vaginitis 616.10
☐ Well Baby/Child V20.2
☐ Weight Loss 783.21
☐ Otitis Media 382.9

Physician's Signature: _____ Next Appointment _____

Instructions: _____

PETTY CASH RECONCILIATION

Period from: _____ to: _____ Department _____

STARTING BALANCE: _____

Date	Petty Cash Voucher No.	Paid to	Charge to	Approved by	Total	Balance
_____	_____	_____	_____	_____	_____	_____
_____	_____	_____	_____	_____	_____	_____
_____	_____	_____	_____	_____	_____	_____
_____	_____	_____	_____	_____	_____	_____
_____	_____	_____	_____	_____	_____	_____
_____	_____	_____	_____	_____	_____	_____
_____	_____	_____	_____	_____	_____	_____
_____	_____	_____	_____	_____	_____	_____
_____	_____	_____	_____	_____	_____	_____
_____	_____	_____	_____	_____	_____	_____
_____	_____	_____	_____	_____	_____	_____
_____	_____	_____	_____	_____	_____	_____
_____	_____	_____	_____	_____	_____	_____
_____	_____	_____	_____	_____	_____	_____
_____	_____	_____	_____	_____	_____	_____
_____	_____	_____	_____	_____	_____	_____
_____	_____	_____	_____	_____	_____	_____

TOTAL VOUCHERS [   ]   [   ]

PETTY CASH REIMBURSEMENT [   ]

BALANCE BROUGHT FORWARD [   ]

Auditor: _____
Date: _____
Over/Short: _____

Approval: _____
Date: _____

Keep in the petty cash box. Reconcile and post to accounts payable monthly.

PETTY CASH VOUCHER

PETTY CASH VOUCHER

Number: _____
Date: _____

For Whom: Amount:

For What:

Acct #:   TOTAL

Approved _____
Received _____

PETTY CASH VOUCHER

Number: _____
Date: _____

For Whom: Amount:

For What:

Acct #:   TOTAL

Approved _____
Received _____

PETTY CASH VOUCHER

Number: _____
Date: _____

For Whom: Amount:

For What:

Acct #:   TOTAL

Approved _____
Received _____

PETTY CASH VOUCHER

Number: _____
Date: _____

For Whom: Amount:

For What:

Acct #:   TOTAL

Approved _____
Received _____

RECEIPT

RECEIPT _____

Receipt Number: _____

Received from:_____
      Address: _____
         For: _____
      _____ Dollars_____

Date: _____   ☐ Check ☐ Cash
Rec'd by:_____   ☐ Credit Card

RECEIPT _____

Receipt Number: _____

Received from:_____
      Address: _____
         For: _____
      _____ Dollars_____

Date: _____   ☐ Check ☐ Cash
Rec'd by:_____   ☐ Credit Card

RECEIPT _____

Receipt Number: _____

Received from:_____
      Address: _____
         For: _____
      _____ Dollars_____

Date: _____   ☐ Check ☐ Cash
Rec'd by:_____   ☐ Credit Card

RECEIPT _____

Receipt Number: _____

Received from:_____
      Address: _____
         For: _____
      _____ Dollars_____

Date: _____   ☐ Check ☐ Cash
Rec'd by:_____   ☐ Credit Card

RECEIPT _____

Receipt Number: _____

Received from:_____
      Address: _____
         For: _____
      _____ Dollars_____

Date: _____   ☐ Check ☐ Cash
Rec'd by:_____   ☐ Credit Card

RECEIPT _____

Receipt Number: _____

Received from: _____
      Address: _____
         For: _____
      _____ Dollars_____

Date: _____   ☐ Check ☐ Cash
Rec'd by:_____   ☐ Credit Card

226

STATEMENT

Account Name: Date:_____

Date:		Amount
	Previous balance	
	Payment received	

PLEASE PAY THIS AMOUNT

A simple statement for a small, non-computerized practice.

TREATMENT ESTIMATE

_____
_____
_____
_____
_____
_____
_____
_____

Other: _____

Other: _____

Total

_____

This is an estimate based on information gained from our examination. If additional problems arise as treatment progresses, this estimate may have to be revised. You will be informed before any unexpected treatment is undertaken. This estimate will be honored for a period of three months only from this date.

Payment Agreement

_____ Treatment estimate

_____ Insurance estimate

_____ Estimated balance

_____ Bookkeeping discount for full payment in advance

_____ Paid now

_____ Due at beginning of treatment

_____ Due at completion of treatment

_____ Remaining balance is payable _____ monthly installments each.

_____ The first installment is due on (date) _____, and

subsequent installments on the same day of each consecutive month.

I have reviewed and approved the above treatment estimate, payment agreement, and terms and conditions on the reverse side and understand that I (patient or parent) am fully responsible for the total payment not covered by insurance.

Date: _____ Signed: _____

Patient (or parent, if patient is a minor)

WAIVER OF PAYMENT DUE TO ECONOMIC HARDSHIP

Patient Name _____

Street Address _____ Phone _____

City _____ State _____ ZIP _____

Medical Insurance Coverage

Company Name _____ ID Number _____

Company Name _____ ID Number _____

I am unable to pay the unreimbursed medical charges due to economic hardship.

Reason:

_____   _____
            Signature   Date

I waive the collection of unreimbursed medical charges on the above-mentioned patient/family. This waiver automatically expires after a period of _____ months unless renewed by me. This waiver may be immediately revoked by the undersigned without prior notice.

_____   _____
        Physician Signature   Date

_____   _____
            Witness   Date

Routine waivers of copayments are illegal for Medicare and for all plans in certain states. If you waive copays for hardship, use this form for audit defense.

WORKSHEET FOR DIVISION OF EXPENSES IN A MULTIDOCTOR PRACTICE

C = Divide by Collections	D = Divide by Doctor (or Department [Dep])
P = Divide by Charges/Production	E = Divide by a Pre-agreed upon *Employee Share Formula*
S = Shared, Amt to Be Negotiated	NA = Not Applicable

Fixed Expenses Occurring Monthly

	Method	Notes
Accounting		
Bookkeeping		
Patient Billing		
Payroll Service		
Auto Expense		
Auto Lease		
Gas, Oil, Maintenance		
Insurance		
Contributions		
Equipment Leases (lease vs. own)		
Computer		
Copier Exp		
-purchase		
-paper		
-supplies		
-repair/maintenance		
Postage Meter Costs		
Clinical Equipment		
Telephone		
Typewriter		
-supplies		
-repair/maintenance		
Insurance		
Major Medical		
Individual (doctors)		
Management Consultants		
Initial		
Ongoing Maintenance		
Marketing		
Telephone Book		
Incentive Thank You gifts		
Practice prom. (entertainment)		
Parking		
Doctor and Staff		
Shared Staff		
Pension/Profit Sharing Contr.		
Doctor		
Staff		
Plant Maintenance		
Office clearning		
Windows		
Plant Care		
Building Exterior		

Many groups, when forming, begin with a very detailed analysis like this to maximize accuracy. They often simplify it later. Accounting must be put on a computerized accounts payable program or spreadsheet. Invite your CPA to sit in on this meeting to fill in this chart.

Method | Notes

	Method	Notes
Rent		
Subscriptions (Recept. Rm.)		
Professional		
Merchant Disc. Fees		
Taxes		
City Business Tax		
City Pers. Prop. Tax		
City Unsec. Pers. Prop. Tax		
Federal Income Tax		
State Franchise Tax		
Other		
Temporary Help—Doctor		
Staff		
Answering Service		

Irregular/Unpredictable Expenses

	Method	Notes
Equipment Repair		
Auto		
Continuing Education		
Doctor (spouse)		
Managerial (?)		
Clinical		
Staff—Managerial		
Clinical		
Hiring		
Advertising		
Agency Fees		
Outside Prof. Serv.		
Temp. Help—emergency		
Other		
Signage		
Petty Cash/Change		

Expenses That Can Increase with Production

	Method	Notes
Collection Expenses		
Small Claims Court		
Clinical Supplies		
Back Off/Clinical		
Table Paper		
Toilet Paper		
Lab Fees		
Office Supplies		
Stationery		
Practice Brochure		
Misc. Supplies and Charts		

	Method	Notes
Salaries		
Doctors (draw)		
Staff		
Shared Staff		
Taxes—Payroll		
Uniforms		
Utilities—Water, Gas		
Elec. Refuse (in rent)		
Postage		
Telephone		
Dictation		

Fixed Expenses Occurring Regularly but not Monthly

	Method	Notes
Accounting		
Tax Preparation—bus.		
Tax Preparation—pers.		
Conventions		
State—Regis. Fees		
Hotel and Travel		
National—Regis. Fees		
Hotel and Travel		
Regional—Regis. Fees		
Dues		
National, State, and Local		
Other		
Insurance (overhead)		
Profess. Property—Comp.		
Fire		
Liab		
Theft/Damage		
Profess. Liability		
Disability—Doctor		
Office Overhead		
Worker's Comp.		
Worker's Comp. Audit		
Life/Disab. Ins. on Debt		
Practice Preservation?		
Licenses		
Clinical		
City, State, and Local		
Marketing		
Quarterly Communications		
Newsletters (Quarterly)		

Other/Miscellaneous Expenses

	Method	Notes

238

HIPAA Forms_____

Introduction

This section contains forms related to the <u>H</u>ealth <u>I</u>nsurance <u>P</u>ortability and <u>A</u>ccountability <u>A</u>ct of 1996 (HIPAA). HIPAA was signed into law in August 1996. The purpose of the legislation was to provide protections on health insurance for an estimated 25 million Americans who move from one job to another, who are self-employed, or who have pre-existing medical conditions. It is designed to improve the availability of health insurance to working families and their children.

As a provider of medical services, you must be aware of your HIPAA responsibilities to secure and protect confidential patient records and information. You must comply with the administrative simplification portion of the legislation which requires that you incorporate HIPAA mandated code sets, forms, policies and procedures into transactions between and among health care providers and payers.

This section includes sample forms such as a Notice of Privacy Practices for Protected Health Information, a Business Associate Agreement, and a Chain of Trust Agreement among others. You can use these forms as templates to create customized HIPAA compliant forms for your office.

AMA SAMPLE PATIENT AUTHORIZATION FORM "A"

Authorization for Use or Disclosure of Information for Purposes Requested by Physician's Office

I, _____[Patient Name]_____, hereby authorize _____[Practice Name]_____: to (check those that apply):

_____ use the following protected health information; and/or

_____ disclose the following protected health information to: _[Name of entity to receive information]_

_____

_____

[Specifically describe the information to be used or disclosed including, but not limited to, meaningful descriptors such as: date of service, type of service provided, level of detail to be released, origin of information, etc.]

This protected health information is being used or disclosed for the following purposes: (be specific)

_____

_____

_____

This authorization shall be in force and effect until _____[specify (1) date or (2) event that relates to the patient or the purpose of the use or disclosure]_____ at which time this authorization to use or disclose this protected health information expires.

I understand that I have the right to revoke this authorization, in writing, at any time by sending such written notification to _[Name of Privacy Contact]___ at ____[Office Address or E-mail Address]___.

I understand that a revocation is not effective to the extent that ____[Name of Practice]_____ has relied on the use or disclosure of the protected health information.

I understand that information used or disclosed pursuant to this authorization may be subject to redisclosure by the recipient and may no longer be protected by federal or state law.

_____[Name of Practice]_____ will not condition my treatment, payment, enrollment in a health plan or eligibility for benefits (if applicable) on whether I provide authorization for the requested use or disclosure.

242

I understand that I have the right to:

- Inspect or copy the protected health information to be used or disclosed as permitted under federal law (or state law to the extent the state law provides greater access rights.)

- Refuse to sign this authorization.

The use or disclosure requested under this authorization will result in direct or indirect remuneration to _____[Name of Practice]____ from a third party (if applicable).

_____   _____
Signature of Patient or Patient Representative   Date

_____
Name of Patient or Personal Representative

_____
Description of Personal Representative's Authority

244

HIPAA PRIVACY AUTHORIZATION FOR USE AND DISCLOSURE OF PERSONAL HEALTH INFORMATION

This authorization is prepared pursuant to the requirements of the Health Insurance Portability and Accountability Act of 1996 (P.L. 104-191), 42 U.S.C. Section 1320d, et. seq., and regulations promulgated thereunder, as amended from time to time (collectively referred to as "HIPAA").

This authorization affects your rights in the privacy of your personal health care information (PHI). Please read it carefully before signing.

_____, ("Covered Entity") will not condition treatment payment, enrollment in a health plan, or eligibility for benefits, as applicable, on your providing authorization for the requested use or disclosure. YOU MAY REFUSE TO SIGN THIS AUTHORIZATION.

By signing this authorization you acknowledge and agree that Covered Entity may use or disclose _____ [describe information] for the purpose(s) of _____ [describe intended use].

By signing this authorization you agree that Covered Entity or its Business Associates may disclose your personal health care information to _____ [identify intended recipients].

Further, by signing this authorization you acknowledge that you have been provided a copy of and have read and understand Covered Entity's HIPAA Privacy Notice containing a complete description of your rights, and the permitted uses and disclosures, under HIPAA. While Covered Entity has reserved the right to change the terms of its Privacy Notice, copies of the Privacy Notice as amended are available from Covered Entity at any of its offices or by sending a written request with return address to _____ [Covered Entity's address].

In accordance with your rights under, and subject to certain restrictions imposed by, HIPAA, you may inspect or copy your PHI in the designated record set maintained by Covered Entity for as long as the PHI is maintained in the designated record set.

You have the right to revoke this authorization, in writing, at any time, except to the extent that Covered Entity has taken action in reliance on it. A revocation is effective upon receipt by Covered Entity of a written request to revoke and a copy of the executed authorization form to be revoked at the address listed above.

This authorization shall expire upon the earlier occurrence of: (a) revocation of the authorization; (b) a finding by the Secretary of the U.S. Department of Health and Human Services, Office of Civil Rights that this authorization is not in compliance with requirements of HIPAA; (c) complete satisfaction of the purposes for which this authorization was originally obtained, to be determined in the reasonable discretion of Covered Entity; or (d) six years from the date this authorization was executed.

By signing this authorization you acknowledge and agree that any information used or disclosed pursuant to this authorization could be at risk for redisclosure by the recipient and no longer protected under HIPAA.

Covered Entity will provide _____ [name of patient] with a copy of this signed authorization.

Acknowledged and agreed to by:

      PATIENT:

By_____   _____
Print Name_____   Date

Address:_____
                _____
                _____

or, ON BEHALF OF PATIENT

By_____   _____
Print Name_____   Date
As_____

Address:_____
                _____
                _____

RESTRICTION OF USE OR DISCLOSURE OF PROTECTED HEALTH INFORMATION (PHI) FORM

I, _____, request that _____[Practice Name]_____

restrict the use or disclosure of my health information for payment or health care operations in the

manner described here: (Please be specific)

_____

_____

_____

I understand that _____[Practice Name]_____is not required by law to accept my

requested restrictions, but if the practice does, _____[Practice Name]_____ agrees to

abide by the restrictions except in emergency situations.

I understand that either I or _____[Practice Name]_____may terminate this restriction in

writing at any time in the future.

Patient Signature: _____

Printed Name and date of birth:_____

Date: _____

Privacy Officer Comments:

____ Accept this request.

____ Reject this request. Reason:_____

____ Patient contacted.

Copy this onto your office letterhead or print it out with your office information typed in at the top.

250

ACCOUNTING OF NON-AUTHORIZED USE OR DISCLOSURE REQUEST FORM

I, _____, request that _____[Practice Name]_____ provide me with an accounting of any and all applicable "non-authorized" uses and disclosures of my protected health information (PHI) between _____ (beginning date) and _____(ending date).

I would like to limit this request for accounting to include disclosures only pertaining to:
_____

I understand that I may be charged for this information if I have previously requested this information within the last 12 months. I have been informed of the approximate cost of $_____, and agree to be financially responsible for this charge.

Patient signature: _____

Printed name and date of birth:_____

Date: _____

Privacy Officer Action/Comments:

Action must be taken within 60 days of the receipt of the request

_____ Request approved

_____ Request denied for the following reason. Health Information was released:

_____For treatment, payment, or health care operations

_____To you

_____With your authorization

_____For National Security Purposes

_____For Law Enforcement purposes

_____As part of a limited data set

_____Prior to April 14, 2003

_____Incident to an otherwise permitted use or disclosure

_____ Request 30-day extension to respond due to _____

_____

Copy this onto your office letterhead or print it out with your office information typed in at the top.

CONFIDENTIAL COMMUNICATIONS REQUEST FORM

I,_____, request confidential communication of my health information when my health information is disclosed on my behalf.

Please use the following address or manner in disclosing my health information to me. (Please be as specific as possible.)

_____

_____

_____

_____

_____

_____

_____

_____ My initials here affirm that failure to disclose my health information in the non-conforming manner stated above could endanger me.

Patient Signature _____

Date _____

Printed Name and Date of Birth _____

Effective Date _____

Practice's Response to Request

_____ Agrees to entire request.

_____ Denies part of requested action because: _____

_____

_____

_____ Requires more complete/specific information to assess your request.

_____ The practice cannot reasonably accommodate your request.

Signed _____

Date _____

Copy this onto your office letterhead or print it out with your office information typed in at the top.

PATIENT ACCESS TO THE MEDICAL RECORD REQUEST FORM

I, _____, request access to my medical records for my personal inspection or by _____, my personal representative. (Please request date and time requested for record access)

Date_____ Time_____

OR

I, _____, request _____[Practice Name]_____ make copies of my medical records for my personal inspection. I understand that these records contain protected health information (PHI). I agree to be responsible for the cost of copying these records, including copying fees, labor, supplies, and postage (if applicable). The charge for this will be $___ per page* and I will be charged a minimum of $_____. I agree to pay for this prior to the service being rendered.

Patient Signature _____

Patient Printed Name and Date of Birth _____

Date of request _____

_____

Practice Response to Request (Must be within 60 days of receipt of request.)

_____ Grants all or part of your request_____

_____ Denies all or part of your request_____

_____

For the following reason: (Circle all that apply)

Not part of your designated record set; contains psychotherapy notes; information was compiled for civil, criminal or administrative actions; subject to CLIA; regards inmate at correctional institution; was created during research; is subject to Federal privacy act; was not created by this practice.

Patient may not appeal if denial is for any of the above reasons

_____ Denied at the discretion of the practice as the information may be harmful to the patient or a third party

_____ Requests a 30-day extension to respond due to _____

Many states have laws that govern how much you may charge for the copying of medical records. Please consult your state laws prior to assessing any fees for copying records.

Copy this onto your office letterhead or print it out with your office information typed in at the top.

PRIVACY COMPLAINT FORM

I, _____, would like to make a complaint about the privacy practices and/or procedures at _____[Medical Practice Name]_____. The following is my statement: *(Please include specific details such as specific personnel involved and the date and location of the event of concern to you.)*

_____

_____

_____

_____

_____

_____

_____

_____

_____

_____

Signature of patient: _____

Date: _____

Copy this onto your office letterhead or print it out with your office information typed in at the top.

NOTICE OF PRIVACY PRACTICES FOR PROTECTED HEALTH INFORMATION

THIS NOTICE DESCRIBES HOW MEDICAL INFORMATION ABOUT YOU MAY BE USED AND DISCLOSED AND HOW YOU CAN GET ACCESS TO THIS INFORMATION. PLEASE REVIEW IT CAREFULLY!

Our office is permitted by federal privacy laws to make uses and disclosures of your health information for purposes of treatment, payment, and health care operations. Protected health information is the information we create and obtain in providing our services to you. Such information may include documenting your symptoms, examination and test results, diagnoses, treatment, and applying for future care or treatment. It also includes billing documents for those services.

[Provider Note: You must include at least one example of use or disclosure for treatment, payment, and healthcare operations, but you may provide more than one example. The examples below are suggestions and should be edited/or replaced to apply to the circumstances of your health care practice.]

Examples of uses of your health information for treatment purposes are:

- A nurse obtains treatment information about you and records it in a health record.

- During the course of your treatment, the physician determines he/she will need to consult with another specialist in the area. He/she will share the information with such specialist and obtain his/her input.

Example of use of your health information for payment purposes:

- We submit requests for payment to your health insurance company. The health insurance company or business associate helping us obtain payment requests information from us regarding the medical care given. _____[Practice Name]_____ will provide information to them about you and the care given.

Example of Use of Your Information for Health Care Operations:

We may obtain services from business associates such as quality assessment, quality improvement, outcome evaluation, protocol and clinical guidelines development, training programs, credentialing, medical review, legal services, and insurance. _[Practice Name]_ will share information about you with such business associates as necessary to obtain these services.

Your Health Information Rights

The health and billing records we maintain are the physical property of the doctor's office. You have the following rights with respect to your Protected Health Information

1. Request a restriction on certain uses and disclosures of your health information by delivering the request in writing to our office—we are not required to grant the request but _[Practice Name]_ will comply with any request granted;

260

2.   Obtain a paper copy of the Notice of Privacy Practices for Protected Health Information ("Notice") by making a request at our office;

3.   Right to inspect and copy your health record and billing record—you may exercise this right by delivering the request in writing to our office using the form we provide to you upon request; appeal a denial of access to your protected health information except in certain circumstances;

4.   Right to request that your health care record be amended to correct incomplete or incorrect information by delivering a written request to our office using the form we provide to you upon request. (The physician or other health care provider is not required to make such amendments); you may file a statement of disagreement if your amendment is denied, and require that the request for amendment and any denial be attached in all future disclosures of your protected health information;

5.   Right to receive an accounting of disclosures of your health information as required to be maintained by law by delivering a written request to our office using the form we provide to you upon request. An accounting will not include internal uses of information for treatment, payment, or operations, disclosures made to you or made at your request, or disclosures made to family members or friends in the course of providing care;

6.   Right to confidential communication by requesting that communication of your health information be made by alternative means or at an alternative location by delivering the request in writing to our office using the form we give you upon request; and,

If you want to exercise any of the above rights, please contact _____[insert name of designated staff member, phone number, or address]_____, in person or in writing, during normal hours. S[he] will provide you with assistance on the steps to take to exercise your rights.

You have the right to review this Notice before signing the consent authorizing use and disclosure of your protected health information for treatment, payment, and health care operations purposes.

Our Responsibilities

The office is required to:

- Maintain the privacy of your health information as required by law;

- Provide you with a notice as to our duties and privacy practices as to the information we collect and maintain about you;

- Abide by the terms of this Notice;

- Notify you if we cannot accommodate a requested restriction or request;

- Accommodate your reasonable requests regarding methods to communicate health information with you; and

- Accommodate your request for an accounting of disclosures.

We reserve the right to amend, change, or eliminate provisions in our privacy practices and access practices, and to enact new provisions regarding the protected health information we maintain. If our information practices change, CMS will amend our Notice. You are entitled to receive a revised copy of the Notice by calling and requesting a copy of our "Notice" or by visiting our office and picking up a copy.

To Request Information or File a Complaint

If you have questions, want additional information, or want to report a problem regarding the handling of your information, you may contact ____[insert name, title, and telephone number of internal contact person]_____.

Additionally, if you believe your privacy rights have been violated, you may file a written complaint at our office by delivering the written complaint to ___[list internal staff member]_____. You may also file a complaint by mailing it or e-mailing it to the Secretary of Health and Human Services whose street address and e-mail address is ___[insert street and e-mail addresses]_____.

- We cannot, and will not, require you to waive the right to file a complaint with the Secretary of Health and Human Services (HHS) as a condition of receiving treatment from the office.

- We cannot, and will not, retaliate against you for filing a complaint with the Secretary of Health and Human Services.

Following is a List of Other Uses and Disclosures Allowed by the Privacy Rule

Patient Contact

We may contact you to provide you with appointment reminders, with information about treatment alternatives, or with information about other health-related benefits and services that may be of interest to you. We may contact you as part of a fund raising effort.

Notification—Opportunity to Agree or Object

Unless you object we may use or disclose your protected health information to notify, or assist in notifying, a family member, personal representative, or other person responsible for your care, about your location, and about your general condition, or your death.

Communication with Family—Using our best judgment, we may disclose to a family member, other relative, close personal friend, or any other person you identify, health information relevant to that person's involvement in your care or in payment for such care if you do not object or in an emergency.

We may use and disclose your protected health information to assist in disaster relief efforts.

Opportunity to Agree or Object Not Required

PUBLIC HEALTH ACTIVITIES

Controlling Disease—As required by law, we may disclose your protected health information to public health or legal authorities charged with preventing or controlling disease, injury, or disability.

Child Abuse & Neglect –We may disclose protected health information to public authorities as allowed by law to report child abuse or neglect.

Food and Drug Administration (FDA)—We may disclose to the FDA your protected health information relating to adverse events with respect to food, supplements, products and product defects, or post-marketing surveillance information to enable product recalls, repairs, or replacements.

[Provider Note: Health care providers working for an Industry performing medical surveillance or evaluating whether the individual has a work-related injury or illness may disclose PHI pertaining to the work-related injury or illness to the employer if the employer needs the findings in order to comply with OSHA regulations.]

[A statement to this effect must be included in the privacy postings of such physicians.]

VICTIMS OF ABUSE, NEGLECT, OR DOMESTIC VIOLENCE

We can disclose protected health information to governmental authorities to the extent the disclosure is authorized by statute or regulation and in the exercise of professional judgment the doctor believes the disclosure is necessary to prevent serious harm to the individual or other potential victim.

OVERSIGHT AGENCIES

Federal law allows us to release your protected health information to appropriate health oversight agencies or for health oversight activities to include audits, civil, administrative or criminal investigations: inspections; licensures or disciplinary actions; and for similar reasons related to the administration of healthcare.

JUDICIAL/ADMINISTRATIVE PROCEEDINGS

We may disclose your protected health information in the course of any judicial or administrative proceeding as allowed or required by law, with your consent, or as directed by a proper court order or administrative tribunal, provided that only the protected health information released is expressly authorized by such order, or in response to a subpoena, discovery request or other lawful process.

LAW ENFORCEMENT

We may disclose your protected health information for law enforcement purposes as required by law, such as when required by court order, including laws that require reporting of certain types of wounds or other physical injury.

CORONERS, MEDICAL EXAMINERS AND FUNERAL DIRECTORS

We may disclose your protected health information to funeral directors or coroners consistent with applicable law to allow them to carry out their duties.

266

ORGAN PROCUREMENT ORGANIZATIONS

Consistent with applicable law, we may disclose your protected health information to organ procurement organizations or other entities engaged in the procurement, banking, or transplantation of organs, eyes, or tissue for the purpose of donation and transplant.

RESEARCH

We may disclose information to researchers when their research has been approved by an institutional review board that has reviewed the research proposal and established protocols to ensure the privacy of your protected health information.

THREAT TO HEALTH AND SAFETY

To avert a serious threat to health or safety, we may disclose your protected health information consistent with applicable law to prevent or lessen a serious, imminent threat to the health or safety of a person or the public.

FOR SPECIALIZED GOVERNMENTAL FUNCTIONS

We may disclose your protected health information for specialized government functions as authorized by law such as to Armed Forces personnel, for national security purposes, or to public assistance program personnel.

CORRECTIONAL INSTITUTIONS

If you are an inmate of a correctional institution, we may disclose to the institution or its agents the protected health information necessary for your health and the health and safety of other individuals.

WORKERS COMPENSATION

If you are seeking compensation through Workers Compensation, we may disclose your protected health information to the extent necessary to comply with laws relating to Workers Compensation.

Other Uses and Disclosures

- Other uses and disclosures besides those identified in this Notice will be made only as otherwise authorized by law or with your written authorization which you may revoke except to the extent information or action has already been taken.

Website

- If we maintain a website that provides information about our entity, this Notice will be on the website.

Effective Date:_____[Insert effective date of the Notice]____(*Must be date when first in effect*)

[Provider Note: You should consult your state law to avoid potential conflicts or contradictions with the uses and disclosures defined in this document.]

HIPAA NOTICE OF PRIVACY PRACTICES

Effective Date: _____

THIS NOTICE DESCRIBES HOW MEDICAL INFORMATION ABOUT YOU MAY BE USED AND DISCLOSED AND HOW YOU CAN GET ACCESS TO THIS INFORMATION. PLEASE REVIEW IT CAREFULLY.

If you have any questions about this notice, please contact _____.

WHO WILL FOLLOW THIS NOTICE

- This notice describes our hospital's practices and that of:

- Any health care professional authorized to enter information into your hospital chart.

- All departments and units of the hospital.

- Any member of a volunteer group we allow to help you while you are in the hospital.

- All employees, staff and other hospital personnel.

[List any other hospitals in your system, subsidiaries or other entities that will follow this privacy notice].

All these entities, sites and locations follow the terms of this notice. In addition, these entities, sites and locations may share medical information with each other for treatment, payment or hospital operations purposes described in this notice.

OUR PLEDGE REGARDING MEDICAL INFORMATION:

We understand that medical information about you and your health is personal. We are committed to protecting medical information about you. We create a record of the care and services you receive at the hospital. We need this record to provide you with quality care and to comply with certain legal requirements. This notice applies to all of the records of your care generated by the hospital, whether made by hospital personnel or your personal doctor. Your personal doctor may have different policies or notices regarding the doctor's use and disclosure of your medical information created in the doctor's office or clinic.

This notice will tell you about the ways in which we may use and disclose medical information about you. We also describe your rights and certain obligations we have regarding the use and disclosure of medical information.

270

We are required by law to:

- make sure that medical information that identifies you is kept private;

- give you this notice of our legal duties and privacy practices with respect to medical information about you; and

- follow the terms of the notice that is currently in effect.

HOW WE MAY USE AND DISCLOSE MEDICAL INFORMATION ABOUT YOU.

The following categories describe different ways that we use and disclose medical information. For each category of uses or disclosures we will explain what we mean and try to give some examples. Not every use or disclosure in a category will be listed. However, all of the ways we are permitted to use and disclose information will fall within one of the categories.

For Treatment

We may use medical information about you to provide you with medical treatment or services. We may disclose medical information about you to doctors, nurses, technicians, medical students, or other hospital personnel who are involved in taking care of you at the hospital. For example, a doctor treating you for a broken leg may need to know if you have diabetes because diabetes may slow the healing process. In addition, the doctor may need to tell the dietitian if you have diabetes so that we can arrange for appropriate meals. Different departments of the hospital also may share medical information about you in order to coordinate the different things you need, such as prescriptions, lab work and x-rays. We also may disclose medical information about you to people outside the hospital who may be involved in your medical care after you leave the hospital, such as family members, clergy or others we use to provide services that are part of your care.

For Payment

We may use and disclose medical information about you so that the treatment and services you receive at the hospital may be billed to and payment collected from you, an insurance company or a third party. For example, we may need to give your health plan information about surgery you received at the hospital so your health plan will pay us or reimburse you for the surgery. We may also tell your health plan about a treatment you are going to receive in order to obtain prior approval or to determine whether your plan will cover the treatment.

For Health Care Operations

We may use and disclose medical information about you for hospital operations. These uses and disclosures are necessary to run the hospital and make sure that all of our patients receive quality care. For example, we may use medical information to review our treatment and services and to evaluate the performance of our staff in caring for you. We may also combine medical information about many hospital patients to decide what additional services the hospital should offer, what services are not needed, and whether certain new treatments are effective. We may also disclose information to doctors, nurses, technicians, medical students, and other hospital personnel for review and learning purposes. We may also combine the medical information we have with medical information from other hospitals to compare how

we are doing and see where we can make improvements in the care and services we offer. We may remove information that identifies you from this set of medical information so others may use it to study health care and health care delivery without learning who the specific patients are.

For Appointment Reminders

We may use and disclose medical information to contact you as a reminder that you have an appointment for treatment or medical care at the hospital.

For Treatment Alternatives

We may use and disclose medical information to tell you about or recommend possible treatment options or alternatives that may be of interest to you.

For Health-Related Benefits and Services

We may use and disclose medical information to tell you about health-related benefits or services that may be of interest to you.

For Fund Raising Activities

We may use medical information about you to contact you in an effort to raise money for the hospital and its operations. We may disclose medical information to a foundation related to the hospital so that the foundation may contact you in raising money for the hospital. We only will release contact information, such as your name, address and phone number and the dates you received treatment or services at the hospital. If you do not want the hospital to contact you for fund raising efforts, you must notify _____ in writing.

For Hospital Directory

We may include certain limited information about you in the hospital directory while you are a patient at the hospital. This information may include your name, location in the hospital, your general condition (e.g., fair, stable, etc.) and your religious affiliation. The directory information, except for your religious affiliation, may also be released to people who ask for you by name. Your religious affiliation may be given to a member of the clergy, such as a priest or rabbi, even if they don't ask for you by name. This is so your family, friends and clergy can visit you in the hospital and generally know how you are doing.

To Individuals Involved in Your Care or Payment for Your Care

We may release medical information about you to a friend or family member who is involved in your medical care. We may also give information to someone who helps pay for your care. We may also tell your family or friends your condition and that you are in the hospital. In addition, we may disclose medical information about you to an entity assisting in a disaster relief effort so that your family can be notified about your condition, status and location.

For Research

Under certain circumstances, we may use and disclose medical information about you for research purposes. For example, a research project may involve comparing the health and recovery of all patients who received one medication to those who received another, for the same condition. All research projects, however, are subject to a special approval process. This process evaluates a proposed research project and its use of medical information, trying to balance the research needs with patients' need for privacy of their medical information. Before we use or disclose medical information for research, the project will have been approved through this research approval process, but we may, however, disclose medical information about you to people preparing to conduct a research project, for example, to help them look for patients with specific medical needs, so long as the medical information they review does not leave the hospital. We will almost always ask for your specific permission if the researcher will have access to your name, address or other information that reveals who you are, or will be involved in your care at the hospital.

As Required By Law

We will disclose medical information about you when required to do so by federal, state or local law.

To Avert a Serious Threat to Health or Safety

We may use and disclose medical information about you when necessary to prevent a serious threat to your health and safety or the health and safety of the public or another person. Any disclosure, however, will only be to someone able to help prevent the threat.

SPECIAL SITUATIONS

Organ and Tissue Donation

If you are an organ donor, we may release medical information to organizations that handle organ procurement or organ, eye or tissue transplantation or to an organ donation bank, as necessary to facilitate organ or tissue donation and transplantation.

Military and Veterans

If you are a member of the Armed Forces, we may release medical information about you as required by military command authorities. We may also release medical information about foreign military personnel to the appropriate foreign military authority. [A hospital that is a component of the Department of Defense or Transportation Department should also include the following: "If you are a member of the Armed Forces, we may disclose medical information about you to the Department of Veterans Affairs upon your separation or discharge from military services. This disclosure is necessary for the Department of Veterans Affairs to determine if you are eligible for certain benefits."] [A hospital that is a component of the Department of Veterans Affairs should also include the following: "We may use and disclose to components of the Department of Veterans Affairs medical information about you to determine whether you are eligible for certain benefits."]

275

Workers' Compensation

We may release medical information about you for Workers' Compensation or similar programs. These programs provide benefits for work-related injuries or illness.

Public Health Risks

We may disclose medical information about you for public health activities. These activities generally include the following:

- to prevent or control disease, injury or disability;

- to report births and deaths;

- to report child abuse or neglect;

- to report reactions to medications or problems with products;

- to notify people of recalls of products they may be using;

- to notify a person who may have been exposed to a disease or may be at risk for contracting or spreading a disease or condition;

- to notify the appropriate government authority if we believe a patient has been the victim of abuse, neglect or domestic violence. We will only make this disclosure if you agree or when required or authorized by law.

Health Oversight Activities

We may disclose medical information to a health oversight agency for activities authorized by law. These oversight activities include, for example, audits, investigations, inspections, and licensure. These activities are necessary for the government to monitor the health care system, government programs, and compliance with civil rights laws.

Lawsuits and Disputes

If you are involved in a lawsuit or a dispute, we may disclose medical information about you in response to a court or administrative order. We may also disclose medical information about you in response to a subpoena, discovery request, or other lawful process by someone else involved in the dispute, but only if efforts have been made to tell you about the request or to obtain an order protecting the information requested.

Law Enforcement

We may release medical information if asked to do so by a law enforcement official:

- in response to a court order, subpoena, warrant, summons or similar process;

- to identify or locate a suspect, fugitive, material witness, or missing person;

©2003 Practice Management Information Corp.

- about the victim of a crime if, under certain limited circumstances, we are unable to obtain the person's agreement;

- about a death we believe may be the result of criminal conduct;

- about criminal conduct at the hospital; and

- in emergency circumstances to report a crime, the location of the crime or victims, or the identity, description or location of the person who committed the crime.

Coroners, Medical Examiners and Funeral Directors

We may release medical information to a coroner or medical examiner. This may be necessary, for example, to identify a deceased person or determine the cause of death. We may also release medical information about patients of the hospital to funeral directors as necessary to carry out their duties.

National Security and Intelligence Activities

We may release medical information about you to authorized federal officials for intelligence, counterintelligence, and other national security activities authorized by law.

Protective Services for the President and Others

We may disclose medical information about you to authorized federal officials so they may provide protection to the President, other authorized persons or foreign heads of state or conduct special investigations. [Hospitals which are components of the Department of State should also include the following: "Security Clearances. We may use medical information about you to make decisions regarding your medical suitability for a security clearance or service abroad. We may also release your medical suitability determination to the officials in the Department of State who need access to that information for these purposes."]

Inmates

If you are an inmate of a correctional institution or under the custody of a law enforcement official, we may release medical information about you to the correctional institution or law enforcement official. This release will be necessary (1) for the institution to provide you with health care; (2) to protect your health and safety or the health and safety of others; and/or (3) for the safety and security of the correctional institution.

YOUR RIGHTS REGARDING MEDICAL INFORMATION ABOUT YOU

You have the following rights regarding medical information we maintain about you:

Right to Inspect and Copy

You have the right to inspect and copy medical information that may be used to make decisions about your care. Usually, this includes medical and billing records, but does not include psychotherapy notes.

To inspect and copy medical information that may be used to make decisions about you, you must submit your request in writing to _____. If you request a copy of the information, we may charge a fee for the costs of copying, mailing or other supplies associated with your request.

We may deny your request to inspect and copy in certain very limited circumstances. If you are denied access to medical information, you may request that the denial be reviewed. Another licensed health care professional chosen by the hospital will review your request and the denial. The person conducting the review will not be the person who denied your request. We will comply with the outcome of the review.

Right to Amend

If you feel that medical information we have about you is incorrect or incomplete, you may ask us to amend the information. You have the right to request an amendment for as long as the information is kept by or for the hospital.

To request an amendment, your request must be made in writing and submitted to _____. In addition, you must provide a reason that supports your request. We may deny your request for an amendment if it is not in writing or does not include a reason to support the request. In addition, we may deny your request if you ask us to amend information that:

- was not created by us, unless the person or entity that created the information is no longer available to make the amendment;

- is not part of the medical information kept by or for the hospital;

- is not part of the information which you will be permitted to inspect and copy; or

- is accurate and complete.

Right to an Accounting of Disclosures

You have the right to request an "Accounting of Disclosures." This is a list of the disclosures we made of medical information about you.

To request this list or accounting of disclosures, you must submit your request in writing to _____. Your request must state a time period which may not be longer than six years and may not include dates before February 26, 2003. Your request should indicate in what form you want the list (for example, on paper, or electronically). The first list you request within a 12 month period will be free. For additional lists, we may charge you for the costs of providing the list. We will notify you of the cost involved and you may choose to withdraw or modify your request at that time before any costs are incurred.

Right to Request Restrictions

You have the right to request a restriction or limitation on the medical information we use or disclose about you for treatment, payment or health care operations. You also have the right to request a limit on the medical information we disclose about you to someone who is involved in your care or the payment for your care, like a family member or friend. For example, you could ask that we not use or disclose information about a surgery you had. We are not required to agree to your request. If we do agree, we will comply with your request unless the information is needed to provide you emergency treatment.

282

To request restrictions, you must make your request in writing to _____. In your request, you must tell us (1) what information you want to limit; (2) whether you want to limit our use, disclosure or both; and (3) to whom you want the limits to apply, for example, disclosures to your spouse.

Right to Request Confidential Communications

You have the right to request that we communicate with you about medical matters in a certain way or at a certain location. For example, you can ask that we only contact you at work or by mail.

To request confidential communications, you must make your request in writing to _____. We will not ask you the reason for your request. We will accommodate all reasonable requests. Your request must specify how or where you wish to be contacted.

Right to a Paper Copy of This Notice

You have the right to a paper copy of this notice. You may ask us to give you a copy of this notice at any time. Even if you have agreed to receive this notice electronically, you are still entitled to a paper copy of this notice. You may obtain a copy of this notice at our website, www._____. To obtain a paper copy of this notice, _____.

CHANGES TO THIS NOTICE

We reserve the right to change this notice. We reserve the right to make the revised or changed notice effective for medical information we already have about you as well as any information we receive in the future. We will post a copy of the current notice in the hospital. The notice will contain on the first page, in the top right-hand corner, the effective date. In addition, each time you register at or are admitted to the hospital for treatment or health care services as an inpatient or outpatient, we will offer you a copy of the current notice in effect.

COMPLAINTS

If you believe your privacy rights have been violated, you may file a complaint with the hospital or with the Secretary of the Department of Health and Human Services. To file a complaint with the hospital, contact _____ [insert the name, title, and phone number of the contact person or office responsible for handling complaints. This should be the same person or department listed on the first page as the contact for more information about this notice.] _____. All complaints must be submitted in writing. You will not be penalized for filing a complaint.

OTHER USES OF MEDICAL INFORMATION

Other uses and disclosures of medical information not covered by this notice or the laws that apply to us will be made only with your written permission. If you provide us permission to use or disclose medical information about you, you may revoke that permission, in writing, at any time. If you revoke your permission, we will no longer use or disclose medical information about you for the reasons covered by your written authorization. You understand that we are unable to take back any disclosures we have already made with your permission, and that we are required to retain our records of the care that we provided to you.

CONFIDENTIALITY AND NON-DISCLOSURE AGREEMENT

I, _____, do affirm that I will not divulge
_____[Practice Name]_____ DATA TO ANY UNAUTHORIZED PERSON FOR ANY
REASON. Neither will I directly nor indirectly use, or allow the use of, _____[Practice Name]_____
DATA for any purpose other than that directly associated with my official assigned duties. I understand
that ALL PATIENT INFORMATION, including financial data, is strictly confidential.

Futhermore, I will not, either by direct action or by counsel, discuss, recommend, or suggest to any
unauthorized person the nature or content of any _____[Practice Name]_____ information.

Violation of confidentiality is cause for disciplinary action, including immediate dismissal.

I understand that signing this document does not preclude me from reporting instances of breach of
confidentiality.

Signed _____ Date _____

286

DEPARTMENT OF HEALTH AND HUMAN SERVICES
CENTERS FOR MEDICARE & MEDICAID SERVICES

Form Approved
OMB No. 0938-0626

AUTHORIZATION AGREEMENT FOR ELECTRONIC FUNDS TRANSFERS

Provider/Physician Name	Provider/Physician ID Number

I hereby authorize _____, hereinafter called COMPANY, to initiate credit entries and if necessary, adjustments for any credit entries in error to my ❑Checking ❑Savings account *(select one)* indicated below and the depository named below, hereinafter called DEPOSITORY, to credit the same to such account.

Depository Name	Branch	
City	State	Zip Code
Transit Number	Account Number	

This authority is to remain in full force and effect until COMPANY has received written notification from me of its termination in such time and in such manner as to afford COMPANY and DEPOSITORY a reasonable opportunity to act on said notice of termination.

Name *(please print)*	Title *(please print)*
Signature	Date

CMS-588 (12-92)

PRIVACY ACT ADVISORY STATEMENT

Sections 1842, 1862(b) and 1874 of title XVIII of the Social Security Act authorize the collection of this information. The purpose of collecting this information is to authorize electronic funds transfers.

The information collected will be entered into system No. 09-70-0501, titled "Carrier Medicare Claims Records," and No. 09-70-0503, titled "Intermediary Medicare Claims Records" published in the *Federal Register Privacy Act Issuance*s, 1991 Comp., Vol. 1, Page 419 and Page 424, or as updated and republished. Disclosures of information from this system can be found in this notice.

Furnishing information is voluntary, but without it we will not be able to process your electronic funds transfer.

You should be aware that P.L. 100-503, the Computer Matching and Privacy Protection Act of 1988, permits the government, under certain circumstances, to verify the information you provide by way of computer matches.

According to the Paperwork Reduction Act of 1995, no persons are required to respond to a collection of information unless it displays a valid OMB control number. The valid OMB control number for this information collection is 0938-0626. The time required to complete this information collection is estimated to average 2 hours per response, including the time to review instructions, search existing data resources, gather the data needed, and complete and review the information collection. If you have any comments concerning the accuracy of the time estimate(s) or suggestions for improving this form, please write to CMS, 7500 Security Boulevard, N2-14-26, Baltimore, Maryland 21244-1850.

288

BUSINESS ASSOCIATE AGREEMENT

Definitions (You may use the catch-all definition or use a specific definition.)

Catch-all definition:

Terms used, but not otherwise defined, in this Agreement shall have the same meaning as those terms in 45 CFR 11 160.103 and 164.501.

OR

Examples of specific definitions:

(a)   Business Associate. "Business Associate" shall mean __[insert name of Business Associate]____.

(b)   Covered Entity. "Covered Entity" shall mean __[insert name of Covered Entity]_____.

(c)   Individual. "Individual" shall have the same meaning as the term "individual" in 45 CFR 1 164.501 and shall include a person who qualifies as a personal representative in accordance with 45 CFR 1 164.502(g).

(d)   Privacy Rule. "Privacy Rule" shall mean the Standards for Privacy of Individually Identifiable Health Information at 45 CFR Part 160 and Part 164, Subparts A and E.

(e)   Protected Health Information. "Protected Health Information" shall have the same meaning as the term "protected health information" in 45 CFR 1 164.501, limited to the information created or received by Business Associate from or on behalf of Covered Entity.

(f)   Required By Law. "Required By Law" shall have the same meaning as the term "required by law" in 45 CFR 1 164.501.

(g)   Secretary. "Secretary" shall mean the Secretary of the Department of Health and Human Services or his designee.

Obligations and Activities of Business Associate

(a)   Business Associate agrees to not use or further disclose Protected Health Information other than as permitted or required by the Agreement or as Required By Law.

(b)   Business Associate agrees to use appropriate safeguards to prevent use or disclosure of the Protected Health Information other than as provided for by this Agreement.

(c)   Business Associate agrees to mitigate, to the extent practicable, any harmful effect that is known to Business Associate of a use or disclosure of Protected Health Information by Business Associate in violation of the requirements of this Agreement. [This provision may be included if it is appropriate for the Covered Entity to pass on its duty to mitigate damages by a Business Associate.]

(d)   Business Associate agrees to report to Covered Entity any use or disclosure of the Protected Health Information not provided for by this Agreement.

(e)   Business Associate agrees to ensure that any agent, including a subcontractor, to whom it provides Protected Health Information received from, or created or received by Business Associate on behalf of Covered Entity agrees to the same restrictions and conditions that apply through this Agreement to Business Associate with respect to such information.

(f)   Business Associate agrees to provide access, at the request of Covered Entity, and in the time and manner designated by Covered Entity, to Protected Health Information in a Designated Record Set, to Covered Entity or, as directed by Covered Entity, to an Individual in order to meet the requirements under 45 CFR 1 164.524. [Not necessary if business associate does not have protected health information in a designated record set.]

(g)   Business Associate agrees to make any amendment(s) to Protected Health Information in a Designated Record Set that the Covered Entity directs or agrees to pursuant to 45 CFR 1 164.526 at the request of Covered Entity or an Individual, and in the time and manner designated by Covered Entity. [Not necessary if business associate does not have protected health information in a designated record set.]

(h)   Business Associate agrees to make internal practices, books, and records relating to the use and disclosure of Protected Health Information received from, or created or received by Business Associate on behalf of, Covered Entity available to the Covered Entity, or at the request of the Covered Entity to the Secretary, in a time and manner designated by the Covered Entity or the Secretary, for purposes of the Secretary determining Covered Entity's compliance with the Privacy Rule.

(i)   Business Associate agrees to document such disclosures of Protected Health Information and information related to such disclosures as will be required for Covered Entity to respond to a request by an Individual for an accounting of disclosures of Protected Health Information in accordance with 45 CFR 1 164.528.

(j)   Business Associate agrees to provide to Covered Entity or an Individual, in time and manner designated by Covered Entity, information collected in accordance with Section [Insert Section Number in Contract Where Provision (i) Appears] of this Agreement, to permit Covered Entity to respond to a request by an Individual for an accounting of disclosures of Protected Health Information in accordance with 45 CFR 1 164.528.

Permitted Uses and Disclosures by Business Associate

1. General Use and Disclosure Provisions (You may list specific purposes or refer to another agreement. See examples below.)

(a)   Specify purposes:

Except as otherwise limited in this Agreement, Business Associate may use or disclose Protected Health Information on behalf of, or to provide services to, Covered Entity for the following purposes, if such use or disclosure of Protected Health Information will not violate the Privacy Rule if done by Covered Entity:

[List Purposes, for example: an answering service, taking medical complaints and identifying patient information such as name, phone number, etc., and submitting this to the physician on—call or however they will do this.]

OR

(b)   Refer to underlying services agreement:

Except as otherwise limited in this Agreement, Business Associate may use or disclose Protected Health Information to perform functions, activities, or services for, or on behalf of, Covered Entity as specified in _____[Insert Name of Services Agreement]___, provided that such use or disclosure will not violate the Privacy Rule if done by Covered Entity.

2. Specific Use and Disclosure Provisions [only necessary if parties wish to allow Business Associate to engage in such activities]

(a)   Except as otherwise limited in this Agreement, Business Associate may use Protected Health Information for the proper management and administration of the Business Associate or to carry out the legal responsibilities of the Business Associate.

(b)   Except as otherwise limited in this Agreement, Business Associate may disclose Protected Health Information for the proper management and administration of the Business Associate, provided that disclosures are required by law, or Business Associate obtains reasonable assurances from the person to whom the information is disclosed that it will remain confidential and used or further disclosed only as required by law or for the purpose for which it was disclosed to the person, and the person notifies the Business Associate of any instances of which it is aware in which the confidentiality of the information has been breached.

(c)   Except as otherwise limited in this Agreement, Business Associate may use Protected Health Information to provide Data Aggregation services to Covered Entity as permitted by 42 CFR 1 164.504(e)(2)(i)(B).

Obligations of Covered Entity

Provisions for Covered Entity to Inform Business Associate of Privacy Practices and Restrictions [provisions dependent on business arrangement]

(a)   Covered Entity shall provide Business Associate with the Notice of Privacy Practices that Covered Entity produces in accordance with 45 CFR 1 164.520, as well as any changes to such Notice.

(b)   Covered Entity shall provide Business Associate with any changes in, or revocation of, permission by Individual to use or disclose Protected Health Information, if such changes affect Business Associate's permitted or required uses and disclosures.

(c)   Covered Entity shall notify Business Associate of any restriction to the use or disclosure of Protected Health Information that Covered Entity has agreed to in accordance with 45CFR1164.522.

Permissible Requests by Covered Entity

Covered Entity shall not request Business Associate to use or disclose Protected Health Information in any manner that will not be permissible under the Privacy Rule if done by Covered Entity. [Include an exception if the Business Associate will use or disclose protected health information for, and the contract includes provisions for, data aggregation or management and administrative activities of Business Associate].

Term and Termination

(a)   Term. The Term of this Agreement shall be effective as of [Insert Effective Date], and shall terminate when all of the Protected Health Information provided by Covered Entity to Business Associate, or created or received by Business Associate on behalf of Covered Entity, is destroyed or returned to Covered Entity, or, if it is infeasible to return or destroy Protected Health Information, protections are extended to such information, in accordance with the termination provisions in this Section.

(b)   Termination for Cause. Upon Covered Entity's knowledge of a material breach by Business Associate, Covered Entity shall provide an opportunity for Business Associate to cure the breach or end the violation and terminate this Agreement [and the _____ Agreement/ sections _____ of the _____ Agreement] if Business Associate does not cure the breach or end the violation within the time specified by Covered Entity, or immediately terminate this Agreement [and the _____ Agreement/ sections _____ of the _____ Agreement] if Business Associate has breached a material term of this Agreement and cure is not possible. [Bracketed language in this provision may be necessary if there is an underlying services agreement. Also, opportunity to cure is permitted, but not required by the Privacy Rule.]

(c)   Effect of Termination.

      (1)   Except as provided in paragraph (2) of this section, upon termination of this Agreement, for any reason, Business Associate shall return or destroy all Protected Health Information received from Covered Entity, or created or received by Business Associate on behalf of Covered Entity. This provision shall apply to Protected Health Information that is in the possession of subcontractors or agents of Business Associate. Business Associate shall retain no copies of the Protected Health Information.

      (2)   In the event that Business Associate determines that returning or destroying the Protected Health Information is infeasible, Business Associate shall provide to Covered Entity notification of the conditions that make return or destruction infeasible. Upon mutual agreement of the Parties that return or destruction of Protected Health Information is infeasible, Business Associate shall extend the protections of this Agreement to such Protected Health Information and limit further uses and disclosures of such Protected Health Information to those purposes that make the return or destruction infeasible, for so long as Business Associate maintains such Protected Health Information.

Miscellaneous

(a)   Regulatory References. A reference in this Agreement to a section in the Privacy Rule means the section as in effect or as amended, and for which compliance is required.

(b)   Amendment. The Parties agree to take such action as is necessary to amend this Agreement from time to time as is necessary for Covered Entity to comply with the requirements of the Privacy Rule and the Health Insurance Portability and Accountability Act, Public Law 104-191.

(c)   Survival. The respective rights and obligations of Business Associate under Section [Insert Section Number Related to "Effect of Termination"] of this Agreement shall survive the termination of this Agreement.

(d)   Interpretation. Any ambiguity in this Agreement shall be resolved in favor of a meaning that permits Covered Entity to comply with the Privacy Rule.

296

CHAIN OF TRUST AGREEMENT

This agreement was created for the State of Hawaii, and can be adapted to your state laws.

This Chain of Trust Agreement is made the _____ day of _____ at _____ , by and between HEALTH CARE ORGANIZATION (the "ORGANIZATION") and BUSINESS PARTNER (the "RECIPIENT"). WHEREAS, ORGANIZATION maintains and operates _____; WHEREAS, RECIPIENT performs _____work which requires it to have access to information regarding ORGANIZATION's confidential and proprietary health information that is considered protected pursuant to federal, state and/or local laws or regulations ("INFORMATION"); WHEREAS, ORGANIZATION desires to protect the confidentiality and integrity of the INFORMATION and to prevent inappropriate disclosure of the information; NOW THEREFORE, the parties agree as follows:

1. CONFIDENTIALITY

Any and all INFORMATION shall be kept confidential by RECIPIENT, and shall not, without legal basis to do so and the prior written approval of ORGANIZATION, be made available to any individual or organization by RECIPIENT or used by RECIPIENT for any purpose other than the performance hereunder. RECIPIENT shall require its employees, contractors and agents to comply with the obligations set forth in this section.

In addition, RECIPIENT shall maintain, and shall require that its employees, contractors and agents maintain the confidentiality of all INFORMATION. RECIPIENT shall comply, and shall require its employees, contractor and agents to comply, with all federal and state statutes and regulations concerning confidentiality of INFORMATION, including without limitations, Chapter 323C of the Hawaii Revised Statutes and any regulations promulgated pursuant thereto, as such statutes and regulations currently exist and as they may be amended from time to time. This provision shall survive the termination or expiration of this agreement.

2. TERM

This Agreement shall be effective _____, 2000, and shall continue _____. This Agreement shall automatically renew itself for an additional twelve-month period unless otherwise terminated by either party. In the event that this Agreement is automatically renewed, RECIPIENT agrees to be bound by the Terms and Conditions currently in effect. The confidentiality provisions of this Agreement shall survive indefinitely, even beyond the termination of this Agreement.

3. DISCLOSURES REQUIRED BY LAW

In the event that RECIPIENT is required by law to disclose INFORMATION, RECIPIENT will provide ORGANIZATION with written notice immediately and in advance of the disclosure, so that ORGANIZATION may take whatever action is deemed appropriate.

4. STATE AND FEDERAL STATUTE COMPLIANCE

RECIPIENT shall maintain all licenses, accreditations and approvals customary to its business, and shall observe and comply with all laws, ordinances, rules, and regulations of the federal, state, county or municipal governments, now in force or which may hereinafter be in force. Further, RECIPIENT understands and acknowledges that RECIPIENT has an affirmative duty to be knowledgeable about and

regarding existing laws, rules and regulations that are applicable to the goods and services covered by this Agreement, and how these laws, rules and regulation apply to RECIPIENT's business.

5.   POLICY AND PROCEDURE REVIEW

Upon request, RECIPIENT shall make available to ORGANIZATION any and all documentation relevant to the safeguarding of INFORMATION including but not limited to current policies and procedures, operational manuals and/or instructions, and/or employment and/or third party agreements.

6.   REPORT OF IMPROPER DISCLOSURE or SYSTEMS COMPROMISE 1

ORGANIZATION and RECIPIENT agree to immediately notify all parties within their Chain of Trust of any improper or unauthorized access and disclosure of the INFORMATION, or any misuse of the INFORMATION, including but not limited to systems compromises. ORGANIZATION and RECIPIENT will take all necessary steps to prevent and limit any further improper or unauthorized disclosure and misuse of information. RECIPIENT shall also maintain an incident log of all improper or unauthorized disclosures. At the request of ORGANIZATION, RECIPIENT will make available to ORGANIZATION a copy of incident log.

7.   RETURN OF MATERIALS

Unless otherwise specifically required by statute or rule, RECIPIENT shall upon request, or at the conclusion of the agreement, return or destroy all material containing or reflecting any ORGANIZATION INFORMATION whether prepared by ORGANIZATION or as a result of providing services for which the RECIPIENT has been specifically authorized by ORGANIZATION. In the case of destruction of the material, the RECIPIENT shall exercise due diligence to destroy the INFORMATION in a manner that will render non-retrievable all documents, memoranda, notes or other writings prepared by RECIPIENT, or its representatives, which are based on the INFORMATION.

8.   SUB-CONTRACTORS

RECIPIENT shall obtain written consent from ORGANIZATION prior to disclosure of INFORMATION to any third party. In addition RECIPIENT shall require any third party to execute a CHAIN of TRUST AGREEMENT that upholds the standards contained within this Agreement.

9.   AGENCY RELATIONSHIP

The parties acknowledge and agree that solely for the purposes of Hawaii Revised Statutes Chapter 323C, in providing the services required by the Agreement, RECIPIENT is acting as ORGANIZATION's agent under an agency relationship. As such, RECIPIENT agrees that it shall be bound by Chapter 323C of the Hawaii Revised Statutes and any regulations promulgated pursuant thereto, as such statute and regulations currently exist and as they may be amended from time to time.

10.   TERMINATION

If, for any reason, RECIPIENT fails to satisfactorily fulfill in a timely or proper manner RECIPIENT's obligations under this Agreement or breaches any of the promises, terms or conditions of this Agreement, and having been given notice of and opportunity of up to 5 days to cure any such default and not having taken satisfactory corrective action within the time specified by ORGANIZATION, ORGANIZATION shall have the right to terminate this Agreement by giving written notice to RECIPIENT of such termination at

least seven (7) calendar days before the effective calendar date of such termination. ORGANIZATION may terminate this agreement immediately upon written notice to RECIPIENT if RECIPIENT fails to comply with Section 4 of this Agreement. Without cause, either party to this Agreement shall have the right to terminate this Agreement by giving written notice to the other party of such termination at least thirty (30) calendar days before the effective date of such termination.

11. GOVERNMENT ACCESS TO RECORDS

In Accordance with 42 U.S.C. Section 1395x (v)(1)(I), RECIPIENT agrees that until the expiration of four (4) years after the completion of services pursuant to this Agreement, RECIPIENT shall make available, upon written request to the Secretary of Health and Human Services, (for Comptroller General of the United States or any of their duly authorized representatives) its contract and books, its documents, and records which are necessary to certify the nature and extent of the cost for services agreed herein to be provided.

Further, if RECIPIENT carries out its duties hereunder through a subcontract with a value or cost of $ 10,000.00 or more over a twelve-month period, such subcontractor shall make available, until the expiration of four (4) years after completion of services pursuant to this Agreement, upon written request to the Secretary of Health and Human Services, (for Comptroller General of the United States, or any of their duly authorized representatives) its subcontract, books, documents, and records which are necessary to certify the nature and extent of the cost for the services agreed herein to be provided.

12. ADDITIONAL ACCESS TO INFORMATION

If RECIPIENT significantly alters the INFORMATION provided by ORGANIZATION, ORGANIZATION shall have the right to access the altered information upon written request to RECIPIENT. Such access shall be provided to ORGANIZATION within a reasonable period after receipt of the request and shall be during the normal business hours of RECIPIENT. RECIPIENT shall incorporate changes or amendments to the INFORMATION if requested by the ORGANIZATION.

13. INJUNCTIVE RELIEF

RECIPIENT acknowledges that the remedy at law for any breach by it or the terms of this Agreement shall be inadequate and that the damages resulting from such breach are not readily susceptible to being measured in monetary terms. Accordingly, in the event of a breach or threatened breach by RECIPIENT of the terms of this Agreement, ORGANIZATION shall be entitled to immediate injunctive relief and may obtain a temporary order restraining any threatened or further breach. Nothing herein shall be construed as prohibiting ORGANIZATION from pursuing any other remedies available to ORGANIZATION for such breach or threatened breach, including recovery of damages from RECIPIENT. RECIPIENT further represents that it understands and agrees that the provisions of this agreement shall be strictly enforced and construed against it.

14. THIRD PARTY BENEFICIARIES

Both parties understand and agree that other parties (individuals or entities) who are the subject of the INFORMATION provided to RECIPIENT are intended to be third party beneficiaries of this Agreement.

15. SEVERABILITY

In the event that any provision of this Agreement violates any applicable statute, ordinance or rule of law in any jurisdiction that governs this Agreement, such provision shall be ineffective to the extent of such violation without invalidating any other provision of this Agreement.

16. CONSTRUCTION OF AGREEMENT

The language in all parts of this Agreement shall in all cases be simply construed according to its fair meaning and not strictly for or against the RECIPIENT or ORGANIZATION. The headings preceding each paragraph are for convenience only and shall not in any way be construed to effect the meaning of the paragraphs themselves.

17. HOLD HARMLESS

RECIPIENT agrees to indemnify, defend and hold harmless ORGANIZATION, its directors, officers, agents, shareholders, and employees against all claims, demands, or causes of action that may arise from RECIPIENT's employees, agents, or independent contractors improper disclosure of the INFORMATION and from any intentional or negligent acts or omissions.

18. GOVERNMENT HEALTHCARE PROGRAM REPRESENTATIONS

RECIPIENT hereby represents and warrants to ORGANIZATION that neither RECIPIENT, its shareholders, members, directors, officers, agents, or employees have been excluded or served a notice of exclusion or have been served with a notice of proposed exclusion, or have committed any acts which are cause for exclusion, from participation in, or had any sanctions, or civil or criminal penalties imposed under, any federal or state health care program, including but not limited to Medicare or Medicaid, or have been convicted, under federal or state law (including without limitation a plea of nolo contendere or participation in a first offender deterred adjudication or other arrangement whereby a judgment of conviction has been withheld), of a criminal offense related to (a) the neglect or abuse of a patient, (b) the delivery of an item or service, including the performance of management or administrative services related to the delivery of an item or service, under a federal or state health care program, (c) fraud, theft, embezzlement, breach of fiduciary responsibility, or other financial misconduct in connection with the delivery of a health care item or service or with respect to any act or omission in any program operated by or financed in whole or in part by any federal, state or local government agency, (d) the unlawful, manufacture, distribution, prescription or dispensing of a controlled substance, or (e) interference with or obstruction of any investigation into any criminal offense described in (a) through (d) above. RECIPIENT further agrees to notify ORGANIZATION immediately after RECIPIENT becomes aware that the foregoing representation and warranty may be inaccurate or may be incorrect.

19. ENTIRE AGREEMENT; AMENDMENTS; NO WAIVER

This Agreement contains the entire agreement between the parties with respect to the matters covered by this Agreement and supersedes all prior negotiations, agreements and employment contracts between the parties, whether oral or in writing. This Agreement may not be amended, altered or modified except by written agreement signed by all parties of this Agreement. No provision of this agreement may be waived except by an agreement in writing signed by the waiving party. A waiver of any term or provision shall not be construed as a waiver of any other term or provision.

20. AUTHORITY

The persons signing below have the right and authority to execute this Agreement for their respective entities and no further approvals are necessary to create a binding Agreement.

21. GOVERNING LAW

This Agreement shall be governed by the laws of the State of Hawaii and shall be construed in accordance therewith.

IN WITNESS WHEREOF, the parties have executed this CHAIN OF TRUST AGREEMENT the day and year first written above.

306

SAMPLE (CHIEF) PRIVACY OFFICER JOB DESCRIPTION

This document was created from the American Health Information Management Association (AHIMA) Website (http://www.ahima.org/infocenter/models/privacyofficer2001.htm) and is provided here for your convenience.

Position Title: (Chief) Privacy Officer[1]

Immediate Supervisor: Chief Executive Officer, Senior Executive, or Health Information Management (HIM) Department Head[2]

General Purpose: The privacy officer oversees all ongoing activities related to the development, implementation, maintenance of; and adherence to the organization's policies and procedures covering the privacy of; and access to, patient health information in compliance with federal and state laws and the healthcare organization's information privacy practices.

Responsibilities:

- Provides development guidance and assists in the identification, implementation, and maintenance of organization information privacy policies and procedures in coordination with organization management and administration, the Privacy Oversight Committee,[3] and legal counsel.

- Works with organization senior management and corporate compliance officer to establish an organization-wide Privacy Oversight Committee.

- Serves in a leadership role for the Privacy Oversight Committee's activities.

- Performs initial and periodic information privacy risk assessments and conducts related ongoing compliance monitoring activities in coordination with the entity's other compliance and operational assessment functions.

- Works with legal counsel and management, key departments, and committees to ensure the organization has and maintains appropriate privacy and confidentiality consent, authorization forms, and information notices and materials reflecting current organization and legal practices and requirements.

- Oversees, directs, delivers, or ensures delivery of initial and privacy training and orientation to all employees, volunteers, medical and professional staff, contractors, alliances, business associates, and other appropriate third parties

- Participates in the development, implementation, and ongoing compliance monitoring of all trading partner and business associate agreements, to ensure all privacy concerns, requirements, and responsibilities are addressed.

- Establishes with management and operations a mechanism to track access to protected health information, within the purview of the organization and as required by law and to allow qualified individuals to review or receive a report on such activity.

©2003 Practice Management Information Corp.

- Works cooperatively with the HIM Director and other applicable organization units in overseeing patient rights to inspect, amend, and restrict access to protected health information when appropriate.

- Establishes and administers a process for receiving, documenting, tracking, investigating, and taking action on all complaints concerning the organization's privacy policies and procedures in coordination and collaboration with other similar functions and, when necessary, legal counsel.

- Ensures compliance with privacy practices and consistent application of sanctions for failure to comply with privacy policies for all individuals in the organization's workforce, extended workforce, and for all business associates, in cooperation with Human Resources, the information security officer, administration, and legal counsel as applicable.

- Initiates, facilitates and promotes activities to foster information privacy awareness within the organization and related entities.

- Serves as a member of, or liaison to, the organization's IRB or Privacy Committee,[4] should one exist. Also serves as the information privacy liaison for users of clinical and administrative systems.

- Reviews all system-related information security plans throughout the organization's network to ensure alignment between security and privacy practices, and acts as a liaison to the information systems department.

- Works with all organization personnel involved with any aspect of release of protected health information, to ensure full coordination and cooperation under the organization's policies and procedures and legal requirements.

- Maintains current knowledge of applicable federal and state privacy laws and accreditation standards, and monitors advancements in information privacy technologies to ensure organizational adaptation and compliance.

- Serves as information privacy consultant to the organization for all departments and appropriate entities.

- Cooperates with the Office of Civil Rights, other legal entities, and organization officers in any compliance reviews or investigations.

- Works with organization administration, legal counsel, and other related parties to represent the organization's information privacy interests with external parties (state or local government bodies) who undertake to adopt or amend privacy legislation, regulation, or standard.

Qualifications:

- Certification as an RHIA or RHIT with education and experience relative to the size and scope of the organization.

- Knowledge and experience in information privacy laws, access, release of information, and release control technologies.

- Knowledge in and the ability to apply the principles of HIM, project management, and change management.

- Demonstrated organization, facilitation, communication, and presentation skills.

[This description is intended to serve as a scalable framework for organizations in development of a position description for the privacy officer.]

Notes

1. The title for this position will vary from organization to organization, and may not be the primary title of the individual serving in the position. "Chief" would most likely refer to very large integrated delivery systems. The term "privacy officer" is specifically mention in the HIPAA Privacy Regulation.

2. Again, the supervisor for this position will vary depending on the institution and its size. Since many of the functions are already inherent in the Health Information or Medical Records Department or function, many organizations may elect to keep this function in that department.

3. The "Privacy Oversight Committee" described here is a recommendation of AHIMA, and should not be considered the same as the "Privacy Committee" described in the HIPAA privacy regulation. A privacy oversight committee could include representation from the organization's senior administration, in addition to departments and individuals who can lend an organization-wide perspective to privacy implementation and compliance.

4. Not all organizations will have an Institutional Review Board (IRB) or Privacy Committee for oversight of research activities. However, should such bodies be present or require establishment under HIPAA or other federal or state requirements, the privacy officer will need to work with this group(s) to ensure authorizations and awareness are established where needed or required.

*Insurance Forms*_____

Introduction

Does anyone like dealing with insurance forms? Not anyone I know!

The politicians that keep promising to simplify paperwork with a government universal health care program apparently have never tried to process a Medicaid or Medicare claim, or even been to the post office to register a letter.

Clean claims and data tracking make paperwork flow smoother. The forms in this section were developed to try to make life a little easier for the accounts receivable department, and their interaction with the rest of the practice.

CHART STICKERS FOR AVERY LABELS #5164

Primary Insurance Co. _____ Eff. Date: _____
Ntwrk/IPA/Med/Grp: _____
Prime Covers: _____ Deductible: _____
Primary Care Physician: _____
Hosp: _____ Admit. Auth. No. _____
Lab: _____
X-ray _____
2ndary Ins. Co. _____ Eff. Date: _____
Copmts: (prime/2nd): _____
In-Office Lab: _____ Other: _____

Primary Insurance Co. _____ Eff. Date: _____
Ntwrk/IPA/Med/Grp: _____
Prime Covers: _____ Deductible: _____
Primary Care Physician: _____
Hosp: _____ Admit. Auth. No. _____
Lab: _____
X-ray _____
2ndary Ins. Co. _____ Eff. Date: _____
Copmts: (prime/2nd): _____
In-Office Lab: _____ Other: _____

Primary Insurance Co. _____ Eff. Date: _____
Ntwrk/IPA/Med/Grp: _____
Prime Covers: _____ Deductible: _____
Primary Care Physician: _____
Hosp: _____ Admit. Auth. No. _____
Lab: _____
X-ray _____
2ndary Ins. Co. _____ Eff. Date: _____
Copmts: (prime/2nd): _____
In-Office Lab: _____ Other: _____

Primary Insurance Co. _____ Eff. Date: _____
Ntwrk/IPA/Med/Grp: _____
Prime Covers: _____ Deductible: _____
Primary Care Physician: _____
Hosp: _____ Admit. Auth. No. _____
Lab: _____
X-ray _____
2ndary Ins. Co. _____ Eff. Date: _____
Copmts: (prime/2nd): _____
In-Office Lab: _____ Other: _____

Cut and paste a master"6-up" meaning six forms to a page, then print and peel or cut up. Put a sticker on each patient's chart. Cover with new stickers for change. Especially good for advising doctor of required ancillary providers for managed care contracts.

CHECKLIST FOR INSURANCE CLAIM PROCESSING

All Cases

☐   Patient's name and policy or group number

☐   Physician's name, ID number, etc.

☐   Diagnosis and procedure numbers, charges noted

☐   Date of service noted

☐   Physician signature

☐   Preauthorization

Surgical/Complex/Referred Case

☐   Copy physician's operative report

☐   Simple explanation of physician's report and equivalency code if for unlisted procedure

☐   Referring and operating physician's name and ID number

☐   Preauthorization

If Appropriate/Workers' Compensation

☐   Doctor's first report of occupational illness or injury

☐   Doctor's supplement or final report

☐   Doctor's report of disability status

☐   Routine measurement of upper/lower extremity

☐   Preauthorization

Post for your accounts receivable staff. Clean and complete claims get paid faster.

ELECTRONIC CLAIMS TRANSMISSION CHECKLIST

Date	Company Transmitted to	No. of Claims	Dollar Amount	Transmitted by	Date Confirmation Required	No. Claims (A)ccepted (R)ejected	Date Errors Corrected	Corrected by

Fill out every time a batch of claims is submitted to track payment and accuracy.

INSURANCE COMPANY SUMMARY SHEET

Insurance Company Name	Copayment Required	Preauthorizations Required	Path Lab Required	Radiology Lab Required	Pharmacy Required	

Keep a copy at the reception phone and window to collect copayments accurately. Keep a copy in exam rooms for provider use.

Predetermination Sent	Predetermination Received	Appointment Schedule	Treatment Completed	Sent for Payment	Payment Received	Predet. Expires

INSURANCE PREDETERMINATION TRACKING

Account No.: _____

Patient Name: _____

Home Phone No.: _____

Insurance Company: _____

Contact Person: _____

Special Notes:

Phone Patient to Bring in Form: _____

Date: _____ Response: _____

_____

Initial Exam Date: _____

Appointment Date(s): _____

_____

Claims Supervisor: _____

Office Notes: _____

_____

_____

_____

	date / by
Sent Note	_____ _____
Predetermination Required	_____ _____
Sent	_____ _____
Received	_____ _____
Date Expires...........................	_____ _____
Reviewed by............................	_____ _____
Work in Progress	_____ _____

Date _____ Place into Section

Reviewed by _____

Submitted for Payment............ _____ _____

Date Sent_____ _____

Reviewed by _____

_____

Payment Received/Denied...... _____ _____

Patient Notified and Billed...... _____ _____

Reviewed by Dr....................... _____ _____

....

_____

_____

_____

_____

_____

_____

_____

_____

_____

_____

_____

Amount of Claim _____

Amount of Check _____

Amount of Write-off _____

Keep in an upright 8½-by-11 ledger tray so that you can flip through the top and easily follow up on the progress of predetermination.

INSURANCE RATE SHEET
Payer Contracted Reimbursement (exclusive of copay/deductible)

CPT Codes				

A handy worksheet for manually auditing reimbursements.

INSURANCE TRACKER

Date:

Patient: Amount of Claim:

Insured: Date Billed:

Address: Dates of Services

Date of Illness or Injury:

Employer:

Address:

Group No.:   Social Security or
                                                  Certificate No.:

Diagnosis
1.
2.
3.
4.

Payment is overdue. Please supply the following information on the above-named patient within 10 days to avoid involving the patient and the state insurance commissioner in a reimbursement complaint.

Claim pending because: _____

Payment of claim in progress: _____

Payment made on claim. Date: _____ To whom: _____

Claim denied: (reason) _____

Patient notified: Yes ( )   No ( )

Remarks: _____

_____

Thank you for your assistance.

Filled out by:

Copy onto letterhead and send if no payment is received in six weeks.

LIFETIME BENEFICIARY CLAIM AUTHORIZATION

Name of Beneficiary _____ Medicare No. _____

I request that payment of authorized Medicare benefits be made either to me or on my behalf to _____ for any services furnished me by that physician or supplier. I authorize any holder of medical information about me to release to the Health Care Financing Administration and its agents any information needed to determine these benefits payable to related services.

I understand my signature requests that payment be made and authorizes release of medical information necessary to pay the claim. If other health insurance coverage is indicated in Item 9 of the CMS-1500 claim form or elsewhere on other approved claim forms or electronically submitted claims, my signature authorizes the releasing of the information to the insurer or agency shown. In Medicare assigned cases, the physician or supplier agrees to accept the charge determination of the Medicare carrier as the full charge, and the patient is responsible only for the deductible, coinsurance, and noncovered services. Coinsurance and deductible are based on the charge determination of the Medicare carrier.

_____   _____
Beneficiary Signature   Date

"Signature on file" form needed for claims or appeals. Copy onto letterhead and save.

LIFETIME INSURANCE AUTHORIZATION

Provider name _____

I authorize the release of any medical information necessary to process claims.

I also authorize payments under my insurance programs to be made directly to the above provider for any services furnished to me.

This authorization also permits the release of information by CMS (its intermediaries or carriers) on any UNASSIGNED Medicare claims to the above.

I further permit copies of the authorization to be used in place of the original.

_____
Patient Signature (or responsible party)

_____
Patient Name (or responsible party) (please print)

_____
Date

Sample form for non-Medicare assigned and other insurance payers. Copy onto letterhead.

MEDICARE BENEFITS EXPLAINED

Dear Patient:

The purpose of this letter is to help you understand your Medicare Benefits Part B—Physician's Services.

When our office accepts assignment that means we will bill Medicare for the benefits due to you and Medicare will send us a check for what it will pay. The payment it makes is almost never the whole amount due.

At the beginning of each year you have a **deductible**. This needs to be paid by you for care before Medicare benefits begin. This amount changes from year to year.

You also have a **copayment** at each visit and for many tests. This is true whether or not a doctor is a participating provider. The U.S. government made a law that Medicare patients must get charged less for visits than other patients. The government set the maximum at a percentage of the level the doctor was charging on July 1, 1984. Your payments and benefits work like this example:

$100.00	Doctor's normal charge
$ 60.00	Medicare's allowable charge
$ 48.00	What Medicare pays at 80% coverage (of $60.00)
$ 12.00	Patient copayment (of $60.00)
$ 40.00	Discount uncollectable by doctor

We *must* bill and collect deductibles and copayments or be subject to section 5220 of the Medicare Carriers Manual, which provides for criminal prosecution by the U.S. Dept. of Justice. We are very careful about not overcharging.

The Medicare system is confusing for doctors and patients alike. There have been over 3,000 changes in the rules in the last four years. If you ever have any questions about billing, please call us. We are here to help you get all the benefits you worked for and are entitled to.

Sincerely,

Office Manager

Copy onto letterhead and give to any patient confused about Medicare payment, copayments, and deductibles.

Patient's Name: _____ Medicare # (HICN): _____

ADVANCE BENEFICIARY NOTICE (ABN)

NOTE: You need to make a choice about receiving these health care items or services. We expect that Medicare will not pay for the item(s) or service(s) that are described below. Medicare does not pay for all of your health care costs. Medicare only pays for covered items and services when Medicare rules are met. The fact that Medicare may not pay for a particular item or service does not mean that you should not receive it. There may be a good reason your doctor recommended it. Right now, in your case, **Medicare probably will not pay for –**

Items or Services:
Because:

The purpose of this form is to help you make an informed choice about whether or not you want to receive these items or services, knowing that you might have to pay for them yourself. Before you make a decision about your options, you should **read this entire notice carefully.**

- Ask us to explain, if you don't understand why Medicare probably won't pay.
- Ask us how much these items or services will cost you **(Estimated Cost: ($_____),** in case you have to pay for them yourself or through other insurance.

PLEASE CHOOSE **ONE** OPTION. CHECK **ONE** BOX. **SIGN & DATE** YOUR CHOICE.

❑**Option 1. YES. I want to receive these items or services.**

I understand that Medicare will not decide whether to pay unless I receive these items or services. Please submit my claim to Medicare. I understand that you may bill me for items or services and that I may have to pay the bill while Medicare is making its decision. If Medicare does pay, you will refund to me any payments I made to you that are due to me. If Medicare denies payment, I agree to be personally and fully responsible for payment. That is, I will pay personally, either out of pocket or through any other insurance that I have. I understand I can appeal Medicare's decision.

❑**Option 2. NO. I have decided not to receive these items or services.**

I will not receive these items or services. I understand that you will not be able to submit a claim to Medicare and that I will not be able to appeal your opinion that Medicare won't pay.

_____   _____
Date   **Signature of patient or person acting on patient's behalf**

NOTE: Your health information will be kept confidential. Any information that we collect about you on this form will be kept confidential in our offices. If a claim is submitted to Medicare, your health information on this form may be shared with Medicare. Your health information which Medicare sees will be kept confidential by Medicare.

OMB Approval No. 0938-0566 Form No. CMS-R-131-G (June 2002)

Medicare requires disclosure in writing to the patient before rendering noncovered services. Copy onto letterhead and give to patient.

MEDICARE SECONDARY INSURANCE BILLING

Dear Patient:

We are currently facing tremendous increases in costs, paperwork, and complications with respect to the many secondary insurance policies held by our patients. As a result we must reexamine our situation in regard to billing these insurance companies for you.

We find we are faced with two choices. Because of the increased labor needed, we must either reduce paperwork or increase fees. The patients we surveyed indicated that they would rather do a little paperwork themselves than pay more for their care.

Therefore, we are introducing the use of simple CHARGE SLIPS for secondary insurances on office visits with our Medicare patients.

When Medicare has paid, simply attach the Medicare Benefits Statement with a legible copy of your CHARGE SLIP to your secondary insurance form and send it into your insurance company for reimbursement. Your insurance company will then pay you your benefits directly. We will still bill your secondary insurance for you on all surgeries. Your payment is due at the time of service or at billing.

We are confident that with your cooperation this new system will work and we will be able to continue providing you affordable care.

Sincerely,

Copy onto letterhead and use as announcement to patients that you will not, or will no longer, accept Medicare secondary assignment.

MEDICARE SECONDARY INSURANCE SIGNATURE ON FILE

I request that payment of authorized Medicare Secondary Insurance benefits be made either to me or on my behalf to _____ for any services furnished to me by that physician/supplier. I authorize any holder of medical information about me to release to _____ _____ (name of insurer) any information needed to determine these benefits or the benefits payable for related services.

Patient's signature _____

Print patient's full name _____

Medicare claim number _____

Medicare secondary insurance company name and address:

_____

_____

_____

_____

Medicare secondary insurance policy number _____

Copy onto letterhead and get signed by Medicare patients with secondary insurance.

PATIENT REGISTRATION UPDATE

Name _____

Please Fill in Only the Section Which Pertains to the Change

Address _____
          (Street)   (City)   (State) (ZIP)

Phone H _____W_____ Marital Status M ____ S ____ D ____ W ____

Insurance: Please indicate if change is in   Primary _____

                                          Secondary _____

New subscriber number _____   New group number _____

New insurance company name _____

Address _____

Phone _____

Employer _____   Phone _____

PLEASE SIGN THE FORM BELOW TO UPDATE OUR RECORDS

ASSIGNMENT OF BENEFITS/AUTHORIZATION FOR TREATMENTS: I hereby authorize treatment and authorize the provider of medical services to release information for these services to my insurance carrier for payment. I further authorize that payment of benefits be made to the provider on my behalf or to myself. I understand that I am financially responsible for all charges not covered by my insurance.

_____   _____

Patient or Authorized Representative   Date

ACCIDENT REPORT

Date and time of report: _____

Name: _____

SS#: _____

Witness(es): _____

Date and time of accident: _____

Location: _____

Injuries: _____

Bodily fluid exposure to victim: _____

Victim bodily fluid loss: _____

Reported to Work Comp. carrier: _____

Where was medical care provided?: _____

Who provided medical care?: _____

Describe accident in detail:

Report Filed By: _____

Victim's Signature that report is correct _____

Other: _____

_____

_____

344

INSURANCE PLAN TRACKING FORM

Insurer Name: _____

Plan Name: _____

HMO, PPO, EPO or Indemnity: _____

Billing address: _____

Claims inquiry phone #: _____

Provider relations phone #: _____

Medical director phone #: _____

Website address: _____

Copay
    Office visit: _____
    WellCare, age birth to _____
    WellCare, age _____ to _____
    Lab covered in office: _____
    Lab not covered in office: _____
    Immunization: _____

Deductible:
Capitated/at risk   (Yes/No)

Required facilities and pre-authorization phone numbers
    Hospital: _____
    Imaging: _____
    Laboratories: _____
    Known excluded services: _____
    _____
    _____

Referral Instructions
    Routine pre-authorization (mail/call) _____
    Hand carry to specialist _____
    Services or amount needing pre-authorization: _____
    _____
    _____
    Plan pre-authorization phone #1 person _____
    Use referral list _____

Reimbursement Rates
    Medicine
    Lab
    Surgery

INSURANCE AUTHORIZATION INQUIRY

FROM:

Doctor _____ Date _____

TO:

Insurance Company _____

Address _____

_____

City, State Zip _____

- - - - - - - - - - - -

RE:

Patient's Name _____

Subscriber's Name _____

Identification # _____

Address _____

City, State Zip _____

- - - - - - - - - - - -

Diagnosis: _____ ICD Code(s) _____

Procedure (s) Planned _____

_____

Hospital/Facility to be used _____

[Yes] [No] Hospitalization Needed? If yes, days requested # _____

[Yes] [No] Pathology or radiology report included

Please inform our office as soon as possible regarding:

[Yes] [No] Is the intended surgery covered under the current policy?

[Yes] [No] Is Pre-Hospitalization Authorization needed?

[Yes] [No] Is a second opinion required?

[Yes] [No] Is hospital/facility covered under the current policy?

Authorizing Agent Signature _____ Date _____

Authorizing Agent Name _____ Date _____

HMO BENEFIT COMPARISON CHART

PLANS

BENEFITS	Plan I	Plan 2	Plan 3	Plan 4
HMO MONTHLY PREMIUM				
HMO CO-PAYMENT (PER VISIT) YOU PAY				
MEDICARE PART B MONTHLY PREMIUM				
MEDICARE PART A & B DEDUCTIBLES & COPAYMENTS				
SKILLED NURSING CARE				
URGENT OUT OF AREA EMERGENCY IN/OUT OF AREA WORLD-WIDE				
CO-PAYMENT WAIVED IF ADMITTED TO HOSPITAL				
EYEGLASSES, FRAMES AND LENSES				
PRESCRIPTION DRUG COVERAGE				
DENTAL COVERAGE				
CHIROPRACTIC CARE				
MENTAL HEALTH SERVICES				
HEARING EXAMS				
HEARING AIDS				
DISCOUNT MEMBERSHIPS EXTRA SERVICES				
GEOGRAPHICAL AREA COVERED				
TOLL-FREE NUMBERS				

350

*Managed Care Forms*_____

Introduction

In a recent article I read that about 78% of all the practices in the country now have at least a little managed care to deal with. Here in California many practices have over 80% managed care patients. Managed care comes in many flavors, from simple preferred provider organizations (PPOs) to fully integrated, multispecialty, risk-sharing, capitated health care organizations (HCOs). One pediatric practice we consulted with accepted over 200 different insurance plans! Try to keep track of that many copayments and deductibles!

Forms for managed information in this area are still developing and are subject to much change. Different information has to be tracked for different reasons and different contracts, often in the same practice. The forms in this section try to help you get a perspective on the impact of managed care in your practice.

CAP RATE EVALUATION—PRIMARY CARE

Determining whether capitation rates will cover the cost of care per patient in your existing practice can be illustrated with this example. Risk pool sharing can provide extra profit.

		Variable 1	Variable 2
Average patient base			
Average visits per patient per	x		
Total patient encounters per year	=		
Months per year	/		
Encounters per month	=		
Overhead per month			
Encounters per month	/		
Overhead per encounter	=		
Active patient base			
Mean capitation/patient/month	x		
Capitation equivalent per month	=		
Encounters per month	/		
Capitation equivalent/encounter	=		
Encounters per month			
Copay per encounter	x		
Copay revenue per month	=		
SUMMARY			
Capitation revenue per encounter			
Copay per encounter	+		
Total revenue per encounter	=		
Overhead per encounter	-		
Profit <loss> per encounter	=		
Encounters per year	x		
Profit <loss> per year	=		
Encounters per year @ 3/patient			
Profit <loss> per year	=		

Note that this approach does not take into consideration profit from nonvisiting members or risk pools. If you don't understand those terms, do not sign a capitation contract.

CAPITATION SPLIT FORMULA

Capitation Data _____

Month _____

Capitation Production	% of Total Production and Gross Capitation Income	Capitation Income
$		
$		
$	%	$
$		
$		
$	%	$
$	%	$
Total $	100%	$

No. of Members _____ x $ _____ PMPM = $ _____

Proofed by documentation _____

_____

_____

For in-depth approaches, buy the book *Physician Income Generation and Distribution Plans* from the Medical Group Management Association at (877) 275-6462.

Capitation Production = Charges on capitated patients
Capitation Income = Gross income to doctor as a % of total cap income
PmPm = Per member per month

COST ANALYSIS FOR CAPITATION CONSIDERATION

A. Total patient visits (encounters) per year _____

B. Total patients per year _____

C. Total receipts per year _____

D. Overhead per year (without physician compensation) _____

E. Average receipt per patient (C ÷ B) _____

F. Average cost per patient (D ÷ B) _____

G. HMO/plan copayment per visit _____

H. HMO/plan copayment per patient per year [(A ÷ B) x G] _____

I. Average HMO/plan FFS compensation per patient (E – H) _____

J. Cap rate proposed per member per month _____

K. Cap rate per patient per year (J x 12) _____

L. Estimated number of members needed per physician _____

(see report NEJM 1-14-93 or JAMA 4-7-89 p. 1932)

M. Number of members needed to equal current receipts

{[C – (BxH)] ÷ K} _____

N. Cap rate per month needed to equal current receipts @ L

({[C – (BxH)] ÷ L} ÷ 12) _____

O. Total HMO/plan membership _____

P. Total physicians (full-time equivalent) needed (O ÷ M) _____

Q. Number of physicians in your specialty in your plan now _____

R. Number of physicians needed (   ) or excess <   > _____

For a more accurate approach, see *Actuarian Issues in the Fee For Service/ Prepaid Medical Group*, available from MGMA at **(877)** 275-6462, or contact a medical actuarian firm.

For section O. (Total HMO/plan membership), modify by age/sex demand for your specialty.

MANAGED CARE CAPITATION FEE-FOR-SERVICE EQUIVALENCY REPORT

Year _____   Specialty _____   Doctor _____

Month	Cap Pmt + FFS + CoPay = Total1	Net FFS + FFSE + MGMT Fee + CoPay = Total2	% Diff.	Totl. Diff.
Jan				
Feb				
Mar				
Apr				
May				
June				
July				
Aug				
Sept				
Oct				
Nov				
Dec				
TOTAL				

Cap = capitated
FFS = fee-for-service
FFSE = fee-for-service equivalent

359

FFSE is your total nondiscounted charges. This form allows you to track your capitated reimbursement and compare it with your FFS to see if you are making or losing money on the contract.

MANAGED CARE CONTRACT REVIEW CHECKLIST

Contract Name _____

- ☐ All attachments, addendums, and documents referenced are attached.
- ☐ All verbal representations made to you are referenced in writing.
- ☐ The contract adequately identifies the entities responsible for payment, including all contact information, and you have confirmed it by actual contact.
- ☐ You have investigated plan references with other doctors or administrators experienced with the plan for ease of communication, prompt payment, hassle fact, etc.
- ☐ You have requested and obtained a financial statement or other support information verifying the plan's solvency and financial strength.
- ☐ You have requested and obtained verification that if the plan represents that it has stop-loss coverage and liability insurance, that coverage is in effect.
- ☐ The contract specifies payment of your fees within a specific number of days and a payer incentive to comply, such as interest or penalties.
- ☐ The contract specifies the reimbursement rate in dollars per procedure code, per member per month, for case management or per hour.
- ☐ You know your costs per procedure, per hour, or per member to deliver care.
- ☐ The contract allows a reasonable time to submit claims and has a provision for extension of that time due to unforeseen circumstances (employee termination or fraud, severe weather, computer malfunction, etc.).
- ☐ The contract has a reasonable claims appeal process and you have checked references on how well it works.
- ☐ The contract does not require you to hold them harmless or indemnify them for any action other than your own.
- ☐ The contract does not required you to pay their legal fees in a patient action, dispute, or for any other reason.
- ☐ The contract will compensate you for any activities required other than patient care and claims processing (such as quality assurance or utilization review or directorships) and provide adequate insurance for those activities.
- ☐ The contract provides adequate description of the quality assurance, utilization review, dispute resolution, or other oversight functions, and those functions appear fair and have input from physicians other than those administratively employed by the plan.
- ☐ The contract does not hold you to a standard higher than "a reasonable physician acting under the same or similar situation."
- ☐ The contract does not require you to obtain an unreasonable amount of professional liability or other insurance; nor that you actually meet or exceed the requirement; and the contract does not require that your policy cover the insurer.
- ☐ The contract does not prohibit you from participating in any other plans.
- ☐ The contract does not allow them to use your name in marketing activities without your consent.
- ☐ There is a confidentiality clause prohibiting the plan from making disclosures about you not indicated in the contract.
- ☐ The contract does not require you to alter your hours, cause hardship in selection of physicians or ancillary services, significantly change your billing practices or use of staff, or other make major changes in the way you practice.
- ☐ The contract provides an adequate panel of specialists and ancillary services.
- ☐ The contract allows for your stopping taking new patients without plan withdrawal of existing patients.
- ☐ The contract allows you to bill patients your normal fee for noncovered services, medically unnecessary services demanded by the patient, patient care after termination of contract, and when the plan is unable to pay or fails to pay
- ☐ The contract provides explicit instructions on patient eligibility verification.
- ☐ The contract provides for reimbursement when mistaken patient eligibility is provided by them to you
- ☐ If you are at risk, you understand the risk.
- ☐ Adequate patients or lives will be available to you.
- ☐ If capitated, you will receive fee for service until an appropriate number of lives are provided.
- ☐ If capitated, you know the age/sex/other demographics and are ideally capitated differently for each group.
- ☐ If capitated, the services included are clearly defined.
- ☐ You have attempted to negotiate better terms.
- ☐ Your internal systems are adequate to accept the plan, track data, and provide reports.
- ☐ You and your staff are adequately trained to provide managed care.
- ☐ The contract allows you an "easy out" in case of dispute, inadequate patient volume, or any other reason without penalty and within a reasonable period of time.

Fill this out on every contract you sign.

MANAGED CARE DATA TRACKING WORKSHEET

	Name _____	Month	Year-to-Date	Last Year-to-Date	Goal
1	Total patients seen				
2	Total ambulatory encounters (AE)				
3	AE/patient (#2÷ #1)				
4	Avg #pts seen/day				
5	#Pts admitted to hospitals				
6	Total hospital days of admits				
7	#Total non-admitted pt hospital encounters				
8	#Total hospital encounters				
9	Hospital charges				
10	Total encounters (#2 + #8)				
11	#Work days				
12	#Work hours				
13	#Encounters per hour (#10÷ #12)				
14					
15	Charges				
16	Receipts				
17	Accounts Receivable				
18	Overhead				
19	Cost per patient (#18 ÷ #1)				
20	Cost per AE (#18 ÷ #2)				
21	Cost per encounter (#18 ÷ #10)				
22	Cost per Hour (#18÷#12)				
23	Avg charges per patient (#15 ÷ #1)				
24	Avg receipts per patient (#16 ÷ #1)				
25	#Capitated (cap) contracts				
26	Charges to cap patients				
27	#Cap lives enrolled (member months)				
28	Total cap payment				
29	Average cap payment per life enrolled (average PMPM) (#28÷#27)				
30	#Cap encounters				
31	Cap payment per encounter (#28 ÷ #30)				
32	Total copays and non-covered services payments from cap patients				
33	Risk pool payments and bonuses				
34	Total payment per member per month [(#28 + #32 + #33) ÷ #27]				
35	Fee for service equivalence [(#28 + #32 + #33) ÷ #26]				

Plan Data Tracking

Plan	Charges	Receipts	Copays & Deductibles	#Lives (cap)	Charges as % of total	A/R

*Marketing Forms*_____

Marketing

Marketing is still a dirty word to some physicians. They think marketing is billboards, abrasive ads and shouting pitchmen.

In reality marketing is any activity to increase the flow of new patients to a practice, and to retain existing patients. Patient service, bedside manner, proper scheduling, decent office decor, and polite receptionists are all good marketing. Our marketing consultants find that about 30% of any doctor's practice is "soft," and can easily be taken away by competitive marketing offering something the patients want but are not getting.

If you want to get involved in serious marketing to increase your practice 20% or more, you really need a medical marketing specialist. Otherwise there are many books and periodicals on the topic to study. These forms can help you put your need in perspective, get organized and track results.

MARKETING ANALYSIS

Objectives

Short-Term:
> Less than one year

Long-Term:
> One year or more

Target:

What Does Target Want?

Who You Are:

Analyze Competition:

Budget:

How to Compete:

Plan of Execution:

Your marketing plans are based on your specialty and environment. Fill out a separate page for each target.

MARKETING CALENDAR

FORM M-2

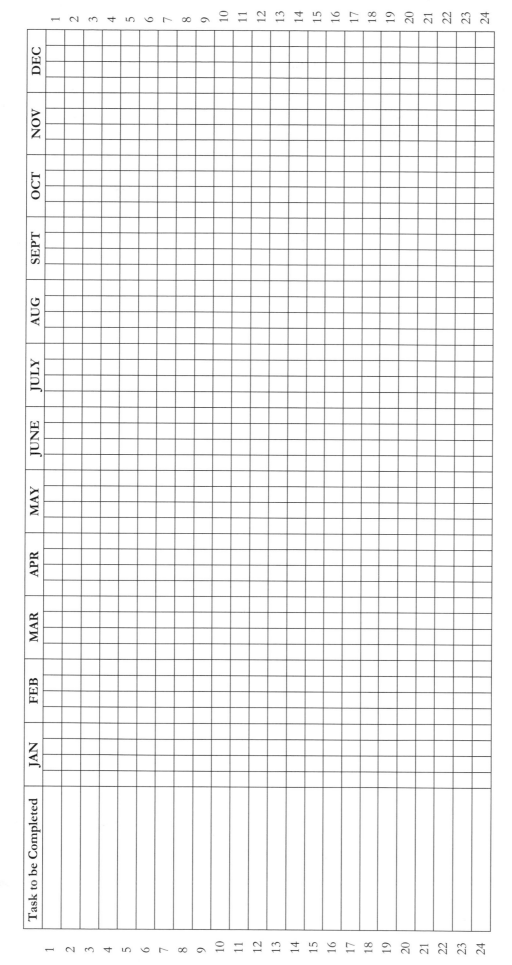

Task to be Completed	JAN	FEB	MAR	APR	MAY	JUNE	JULY	AUG	SEPT	OCT	NOV	DEC	
1													1
2													2
3													3
4													4
5													5
6													6
7													7
8													8
9													9
10													10
11													11
12													12
13													13
14													14
15													15
16													16
17													17
18													18
19													19
20													20
21													21
22													22
23													23
24													24

Try to balance your activities so they don't all crush you at once.

MARKETING GOALS

Goal Receipts/Month _____

Total Receipts/Month Now   (minus)   _____

Increased Receipts Needed   (equals)   _____

Collection Ratio (Receipts ÷ Charges)   %   _____

Increased Charges Needed to Achieve Receipts
    (Increased Receipts ÷ Collection Ratio)   _____

Average Charge per Patient   _____

Number of Patients Needed to Reach Goal
    (Charges Needed ÷ Avg. Charge per Patient   _____

$ Overhead per Patient Now   _____

$ Additional Overhead per New Patient
    (Variable Overhead if Fixed Costs Have Been Met)   _____

$ Profit per New Patient   _____

Marketing Costs Budget per New Patient   _____

Marketing Costs per Month Total
    (Budget per Patient x Number of Patients Needed)   _____

Use this form to do a financial analysis of your marketing plans.

MARKETING SURVEY CHART

1 = Medical Sophistication (Quality)
2 = Cost Leadership
3 = Convenience
4 = Communications
5 = Focus
6 = Service₁

7 = Innovation
8 = Contracts
9 =
10 =
11 =
12 =

	1	2	3	4	5	6	7	8	9	10	11	12
10												
9												
8												
7												
6												
5												
4												
3												
2												
1												
NA												

373

Use this chart to compare yourself with your competitors, and then consider the changes that are necessary.

WEB PAGE PLANNER

Please assemble or write all appropriate components of the following list as it would pertain to the website you wish to have created. The more you prepare, the less it costs. Provide the information to your selected webpage designer, preferably in electronic format.

Target Audience
Featured Product/Service/Specialty
Pitch/hook/call to action
Any special web directories on which you wish this page to be listed

Title (5-10 words) (this will appear in the page Title Bar on browsers)
Description (for meta tag, limit 200 characters)
Keywords (for meta tag, limit 20 words)
Domain name(s) owned or desired
Logos and images available
Images desired
Patient stories
CV
Photo(s), doctor, staff, clinical
Books authored or recommended
Articles authored or recommended
Seminars/lectures (upcoming and done)
News (if you use this category, be prepared to update it at least monthly)
Professorships
Practice description
Philosophy/mission
Board certifications
Awards
Inventions
Practice brochure info:
       appointment info
       email appointments accepted?
       directions
       insurances accepted
       tests and x-rays
       telephone calls
       fees
       self-referral self-evaluation template
       staff privileges at hospitals, surgicenters etc

Note: the authors of this book offer a Web Site Optimization service, applying the latest techniques to make web sites easily findable to searchers. Author Keith Borglum, at the time of writing, is the Editor for Medical Marketing for the Open Directory Project (ODP). ODP powers the core directory services for the Web's largest and most popular search engines and portals, including Netscape Search, AOL Search, Google, Lycos, HotBot, DirectHit, and hundreds of others. If you wish to have your web site optimized, it would be best to contact the authors prior to engaging a webmaster. Authors can be contacted via their website at MedicalPracticeManagement.com.

PRESS RELEASE

Date:
Contact Person:
For Immediate Release: (or Hold for Release Date_____)

Subject: CATCHY TITLE IN ALL CAPITALS

The first sentence and first paragraph is important for presenting the most important or attention-getting facts of the story. Remember "who, what, when, where, and why." The reporter or editor may very well rewrite your release. Use double spacing and wide margins to allow the editor room to make notes. Use left-justify to layout the type.

Use the first or second paragraphs to include the name of the physician or practice, and how it connects to the story. Do not make the press release obviously self-serving. Make it newsy. Taking a local angle to a national story with local facts often works well. For example, "The new studies on hormone replacement therapy indicate that one woman in 2,300 will develop breast cancer due to hormone therapy. According to Dr. Smith of the Smith Woman's Clinic, that means approximately 15 cases here in Anytown."

A quote should be included that is attributable to the physician. It should help establish credibility. Use terms like "said, noted, indicated," not "claimed, declared, or denied."

If you have more information, include it in the fourth paragraph. Quoting the doctor again might be OK. This paragraph might well be eliminated by the editor to save space.

Finish with a recap of major points or recommendations for action. Say, "See your physician if you have questions," not "see Dr. Smith . . ." You can work in your phone number, email address or website here. You can say, "More information is available on Dr. Smith's website at . . ."

It is best to submit your release to the person in charge of health-related articles in the target media. That person is often identified on the media's web page, including their email address and guidelines for submitting press releases. Ask them what kind of stories they are interested in. Putting three #s marks the end of the story.

###

Personnel Forms

Introduction

Staffing is the biggest expense in almost every specialty. It therefore demands the most attention. Finding, hiring, training, keeping, reprimanding, and firing staff is important work. Skipping one step in the process can be disastrous. About 80% of our consulting involves personnel in one way or another.

There are some bad apples out there. It is estimated that about one half of all practices experience staff embezzlement or theft at some time. Our consultants catch a few embezzlers every year. When they get out of jail, they usually get a job with another doctor. Having proper hiring policies will keep them out of your practice.

Wrongful termination, wrongful non-hire, and staff harassment are growth industries for the legal profession. If you use these forms you will reduce your liability significantly. See your attorney to modify them for use in your state before implementing since laws vary widely.

ADVERTISING FOR NEW STAFF

Run a classified ad continuously until one week after the new staff member is hired in order to draw from abundance and in case the person hired does not work out. (You will know in a week.)

If your ad does not attract a strong response in the first week, reevaluate and determine if it is the best ad in its section. If not, change it or change sections. Do not get discouraged and do not settle for second best. You may have to review 50 or 75 (or more) applicants to find the best person, and it could take a month.

When advertising for a business office assistant, have the paper assign a box number and ask applicants to send résumés. Assign a skills "screener" to handle mail inquires (unless you have a lot of time to spend answering the telephone). Review the résumés carefully. You might want to request a handwritten cover letter when recruiting for a front desk position.

Telephone those with appropriate résumés and listen carefully to their voices and verbal skills. If they do not sound good on the phone, do not interview them face to face.

If they sound good, schedule 15-minute interviews with them. If they shine at the interview, reschedule them for a 30-minute interview and have them fill out a job application. Delegate this whole process to a staff person if possible; you should be face-to-face interviewing (for 30 minutes) only the top three applicants.

Check references on your top three.

If possible, have the new staffer come into your office to observe for a half day.

ALWAYS, ALWAYS use specific tests or watch them using their technical skills no matter how many years of experience they have or who refers them to you!

AFFIRMATIVE ACTION QUESTIONNAIRE

Social Security Number   Exact Title of Position

We are asking all applicants for examinations to voluntarily complete this form in order to comply with United States government Equal Employment Opportunity requirements. This information will be detached from this application and will be used for statistical purposes only. This information will have no effect on your application.

Check one only:

☐ Asian/Pacific Islander   ☐ Female   ☐ Male

☐ American Indian/Alaskan Native   ☐ Over 40?

☐ Black   ☐ Under 18?

☐ Filipino   If yes, can you supply a work permit?

☐ Hispanic   ☐ Yes   ☐ No

☐ White

Do you have a disability which will limit your ability to compete in the examination process as described in the job announcement? ☐ Yes   ☐ No

If your answer is yes, please call the Personnel Department at _____ to discuss possible reasonable accommodation. A reasonable effort will be made to assist you.

How did you learn about this examination?

Check on only:

(1) ☐ County bulletin

(2) ☐ County employee

(3) ☐ Job hot line

(4) ☐ Public office other than county

(5) ☐ Minority organization or group

(6) ☐ Women's organization or group

(7) ☐ School

(8) ☐ Other (please specify) _____

_____

Newspaper

(9) ☐ _____

(10) ☐ _____

(11) ☐ _____

(12) ☐ _____

(13) ☐ _____

(14) ☐ _____

Other Publication

(15) ☐ Jobs available

(16) ☐ Other publication (name)

This form need be used only if you are required to by size.

PRACTICE NAME   ADDRESS   PHONE NO.

PLEASE PRINT OR TYPE

Exact Title of Position: _____   Social Security Number: _____

Name: _____   Home Telephone: _____

Mailing Address: _____   Work Telephone: _____

City: _____   State and ZIP Code: _____

Indicate ALL TYPES of work you are willing to accept:

☐ Full time (full benefits)

☐ Part time (less than 40 hours per week—partial benefits)

☐ Extra help (temporary or relief-no benefits)

Is there any department where you are NOT willing to work:

☐ Yes   ☐ No

☐ Where _____

_____

What shift assignments are you willing to accept:

☐ Days   ☐ PMs

☐ Nights   ☐ Weekends

Do you have a valid driver's license?

☐ Yes   ☐ No

State: _____ No: _____ Class: _____

Languages other than English?

	Speak	Read	Write
_____	☐	☐	☐
_____	☐	☐	☐
_____	☐	☐	☐

Affirmative answers to the following questions are not necessarily a bar to employment. Each case is considered in relationship to the requirements for the position(s) for which you are applying. Give detail to any "yes" answers in the space provided below.

If the job you are applying for requires driving please answer this question. Have you ever been put on probation or has your driver's license been suspended or revoked within the last five years?

☐ Yes   ☐ No

As an adult have you ever been convicted of a felony within the last 10 years?

☐ Yes   ☐ No

Please give details for any "yes" responses:

Have you ever been discharged, released during a probationary period, or been requested to resign under unfavorable circumstances from any employment within the last five years?

☐ Yes   ☐ No

Have you previously been employed by us?

☐ Yes   ☐ No

Former employees who were released from probation or had disciplinary actions during the past 12 months are precluded from applying.

_____

_____

_____

PRIVACY STATEMENT AND CERTIFICATE OF APPLICANT
PLEASE READ CAREFULLY BEFORE SIGNING

I understand that the information I provide on this form will be used to determine whether I meet the requirements for this examination only and may serve as the basis for arriving at my final rating. I also understand and agree that providing the requested information is voluntary and that omission or distortion of any item may result in my qualifications not receiving full consideration, may disqualify me from participating further in the examination process, or may result in my termination from employment.

Signature _____ Date _____

FOR PERSONNEL USE ONLY

A_____ R _____
Analyst

_____

_____

_____

EMPLOYEE ATTENDANCE RECORD

FORM P-3

First Name   Last Name   Position

ABSENCE SUMMARY

	A	CE	DF	H	J	LA	P	SS	T	V

YEARLY TOTALS

20__	1	2	3	4	5	6	7	8	9	10	11	12	13	14	15	16	17	18	19	20	21	22	23	24	25	26	27	28	29	30	31	ttl hrs wrkd
Jan																																
Feb																																
Mar																																
Apr																																
May																																
Jun																																
Jul																																
Aug																																
Sept																																
Oct																																
Nov																																
Dec																																

A = absence—no notice
CE = continuing ed
DF = death in family
H = holiday
J = jury duty
LA = leave of absence
P = personal leave
SS = sickness-self
T = tardy
V = vacation

387

Just fill in the absences.

EMPLOYEE HIRING WORKSHEET

Date: _____

Name _____ Interviewer _____

Explain the position to the applicant, then ask questions, and then LISTEN

Ask the following questions of the applicant face to face. Make brief notes as you go on this sheet of paper. Pay special attention to unspoken messages, pauses or hesitations, open and closed body language, etc.

Tell me about your qualifications and skills as you see them for the position I have described:

Why did you apply for this job?

If you could design the ideal job for yourself, what would it be like?

Describe a project, change, or procedure you designed or helped to implement that: 1) helped serve patients better, 2) saved $, or 3) made $ for the _____ you last worked for/with:

What characteristics about yourself do you like the best?

What do you see as your learning areas?

Why did you leave your last job?

What did you like best about your last job? Least?

What motivates you to do an outstanding job?

If your present employer would increase your earnings to the amount you seek, what would you do?

What physical condition do you have which may limit your ability to perform this job?

How flexible can you be in your working days and hours?

May I contact your present employer as one of your references?

Describe your short- and long-term career goals.

What accomplishments, even project, etc., were you most proud of?

Evaluation Key	
4 = needs improvement	
3 = fair	
2 = OK	
1 = excellent	

_____ Personal appearance   _____ Discreet/confidential
_____ Professional conduct   _____ On time for appointment
_____ Speaks clearly   _____ Hygiene
_____ Pleasing personality   _____ Open to learning
_____ Seems truthful   _____ Sensitive, listens, honest
_____ Self-confident   _____ Cheerful, interested

Fill out an interview sheet immediately after the interview. Ask questions, like these, that force the applicant to say more than "uh-huh" or "uh-uh."

EMPLOYEE INFORMATION RECORD

Doctor Name _____

Date _____

_____

Employee

_____

Social Security Number   Position

_____

Street Address   City   State   ZIP Code

_____

Birth Date   Home Telephone

Emergency Information

| | Home telephone |
| | Work telephone |

Person to Contact   Relationship

_____

Street Address   City   State   ZIP Code

I have read and understand the personnel policy: _____

Employee signature   Date

For Office Use Only

Hr/Day/Wk/Mo

Date of hire   Initial period ends   Beginning salary   Circle one

Date eligible for benefits   Type of benefits

Termination   **Date** _____

Reason for separation_____

_____

_____

_____

Letter of recommendation given   ☐ Yes   ☐ No   By: _____

Eligible for rehire: ☐ Yes   ☐ No   By: _____

This form is filled out after the employee is hired.

EMPLOYEE INFORMATION RECORD

Review Date	Rev by Initials	Salary Change/if Appr. From	To	Current Position	CC to Empl	Next Eval Date	Comments

Fill out for every pay or benefit change or review.

EMPLOYEE REVIEW

	Unacceptable	Needs Improvement	Satisfactory	Excellent
Employee Name: _____ Date: _____				
Reviewed by: _____ Empl. Record Update: _____				
1. Personal appearance				
2. Conducts self in a professional manner with patients				
3. Uses language becoming a professional				
4. Performs well under pressure				
5. Communicates openly				
6. Leaves personal affairs at home				
7. Accepts and follows established rules and procedures				
8. Discreet about confidential information, both patient and personal				
9. Demonstrates responsibility for good attendance and punctuality				
10. Performs with minimal supervision				
11. Completes work on time				
12. Makes efficient use of time				
13. Responds to directions quickly				
14. Does share of workload				
15. Organizes work in efficient and practical manner				
16. Has an interest in job and patients				
17. Work is neat and legible				
18. Cooperates and works well with people				
19. Accepts changes in routine and procedures willingly				
20. Puts original and constructive thinking into practice				
21. Can see things to be done and proceeds to do them without being told				
22. Respects other person's opinion even if in disagreement				
23. Takes care of own physical health				
24. Seeks new knowledge and skills				
25. Provides patient education				
26.				
27.				
28.				
29.				
30.				

I have discussed this review with the employee.

_____   _____
(Reviewer)   (Date)

I have read and understand this employee review and received a copy of it.

_____   _____
(Employee)   (Date)

See reverse for narrative and specific notes

395 ©2003 Professional Management & Marketing

Do reviews quarterly for improved communication. Staff can do them on doctors too!

EMPLOYEE REVIEW

Employee Name: _____

Reviewed by: _____ Date _____

Specific strengths: _____
_____
_____
_____

Specific learning areas: _____
_____
_____
_____

Specific changes needed: _____
_____
_____
_____

What specifically will be done?/Goals	By whom	By when
_____		
_____		
_____		
_____		
_____		
_____		

Consequences if not completed: _____
_____
_____

Rewards/incentives if completed: _____
_____
_____

Next review scheduled for: _____ Received: _____

This page is used mostly for reprimands and prefiring documentation.

EMPLOYMENT AGREEMENT

This agreement is made and entered into on (date) _____

between (employer) _____

and (employee) _____

At-will employment with _____

shall begin on (date) _____ and be subject to the written personnel policy.

Employer shall pay to the employee a _____ salary/wage of $ _____ per _____ .
Salary/wage increases, except as noted here, shall be based on merit and employee production.
(Regular reviews will not necessarily or automatically include increases):

_____

_____

_____

_____

_____

_____

_____

Benefits provided are per the office personnel policy, which is hereby incorporated by reference and made a part of this agreement.

Other compensation/benefit issues:

_____

_____

_____

_____

The employee shall perform duties as _____
as required by his/her job description as stated in the office personnel policy and as requested by the employer/supervisor.

In witness thereof, the parties have read, understood, and agreed to this agreement and to the office personnel policy.

_____   _____
            Employer   Date

_____   _____
            Employee   Date

Prepare a written Employment Agreement for all employees.

EMPLOYMENT APPLICATION

Date: _____

Last Name: _____ First Name: _____ M/I: _____

Street Address: _____ City: _____

State: _____ZIP: _____ Telephone No.: _____

Social Security No.: _____

Employment Desired	Position	FT/PT	Date Avail	Salary Des.

Are you employed presently? Yes ☐ No ☐ If so, may we contact your present employer? ☐ Yes ☐ No

Have you ever applied to this office before?　　Yes ☐　　No ☐　　　When: _____

Education	Name and Location of Schools	Did You Graduate?	Subjects Studied
High School		Y/N	
College/s		Y/N	
Trade, Business, Corresp. School		Y/N	

Continuing education or special training (please specify) _____
_____
_____
_____

Experience:
Indicate Years

☐	Typing
☐	Filing
☐	Phones
☐	Scheduling
☐	Insurance Billing
☐	Computer
☐	Collections/Phone

☐	Over the Counter
☐	Collections
☐	Supervision
☐	Accounts Payable
☐	General Ledger
☐	Profit and Loss
☐	Back Office

☐	Injections_____
☐	Venipuncture
☐	BPs, HTS, WTS
☐	_____
☐	_____
☐	_____
☐	_____

Watch out for lines left blank. They may mean something. All applicants should fill out an application even if they have résumés.

Employers
list last one first

EMPLOYMENT
APPLICATION

From	To	Employer	City	Position
		Phone No.	Salary	Reason for leaving

References (Name, Address, and Phone No.)	Business Name	Years Acquainted

Have you ever been convicted of a felony? If yes, please explain. (Use the back of this sheet if necessary.)
_____
_____

I authorize all persons and companies named above and others determined appropriate, excepting my present employer if so noted, to furnish any information regarding me whether or not it is on their records and hereby release them from all liability for damage for providing this information. In addition, I understand that a routine inquiry may be made which will validate the information I have placed on this application. Upon my written request, additional information as to the nature and scope of the inquiry, if one is made, will be provided to me. I further understand that any employment offered to me will not be for any definite period of time and is subject to termination, with or without cause, by employer or at my own election at any time for any reason. I understand that my employment is at will and that this policy cannot be changed except in a written document signed by an authorized officer of the company and also signed by me.

Date: _____   Signature: _____

DO NOT WRITE BELOW THIS LINE

Interviewed by:			
Remarks			
References checked, date:		Neatness:	
Ability		Projected Review Date	
Date Hired	Will Report	Employee information record completed, Date	
Position	Salary/Wages	1st Review Date:	Pers. Pol. Signed, Date

EXIT CHECKLIST

Name _____

Returned the following company property:

	Response	Received (initial/date)

Items

Office keys:
Front/back door   _____   _____
Filing cabinets   _____   _____
Cash box   _____   _____

Manuals (including but not limited to):
Policy and procedure   _____   _____
Lab   _____   _____

All documents and paraphernalia
Forms   _____   _____
Reports   _____   _____
Appointment records   _____   _____
Any and all materials/items related
to the practice: _____   _____
      Pager   _____   _____
      Portable   _____   _____

Responses:

1.   Returned
2.   Not applicable
3.   Destroyed and/or no longer available
4.   Did not return

Provided

Wages   _____   _____
Unused benefit compensation   _____   _____
Retirement plan funds   _____   _____
Severance   _____   _____
Reference letter   _____   _____

- -

As an exiting employee, I understand that any and all patient or practice-related information is to remain confidential.

Employee _____
Date of hire _____
Full time _____ Part time _____
Wage at hire _____ Wage at exit _____
Position at hire _____
Position at exit _____
Exit date _____
Eligible for rehire _____
Reason _____
Employee signature _____ Supervisor signature _____

HOW TO CONDUCT A REFERENCE CHECK

You can use the wording as show below by filling in the blanks with the appropriate information

This is _____ of Dr. _____. _____ has applied for work in our (practice or firm).

May I speak to someone who can verify _____'s employment information?

(If transferred to another person, repeat the first two sentences again)

_____ states that she/he worked with you from _____ (date) to _____(date). If this correct? Yes   No

She/he lists her/his position with you as _____, correct? Yes   No

_____indicated her/his salary was _____ at the time she/he left, is this correct? Yes   No

Did absenteeism present any problems? Yes   No

Was her/his work satisfactory? Yes   No

_____ states her/his reason for leaving was _____. Is that correct? Yes   No

Would you rehire _____ if the position became open again? Yes   No   Hesitation

With whom am I speaking, please? _____

What is your position with the office? _____

Thank you for your help.

* Note: If the office is open to sharing, you can also ask what they saw as the individual's strengths and learning areas.

Telephone number:

Person making call:

Date: Time:

Comments:

_____
_____
_____
_____
_____
_____

Use one sheet for each reference and attach to resume or new employee file

Always check references.

INDEPENDENT CONTRACTOR INFORMATION

To further clarify your independent contractor status for the IRS please read this, sign below, and return.

- You are provided instructions as to how to perform your tasks.

- You may have other persons substitute for you to achieve results.

- You set your own schedule and hours.

- Your work is not essential to the running of our firm.

- You have time to perform other work and do so.

- You control any assistants you hire.

- You decide when and where your work is done.

- You control the sequence of tasks.

- You are not required to submit progress reports.

- You pay your own business expenses.

- You furnish your own "tools."

- You purchase your own letterhead, business cards, etc.

- You operate independently of our facilities.

- Your services are available to others.

- You are not paid for partial completion of a job.

- Your job is paid by agreement.

- You are free to produce results in your own way.

The above confirms our understanding.

_____   _____
Doctor   Independent Contractor

_____   _____
Date   Date

There are serious tax consequences to the "employer" if the IRS disallows independent contractor relationships. If you are treating any persons, including doctors, as ICs and they don't fit the above criteria, see your CPA as soon as possible.

PAYROLL RECORD, INDIVIDUAL

Name: _____ **Social Security No.** _____

No. of Exemptions _____ ☐ **Single**   ☐ **Married**

	DEDUCTIONS				PAY			NET PAY	CHECK NUMBER
Date	Social Security	Withholding Taxes			Insurance				
		Federal	State	Local					

REVIEWING RÉSUMÉS

General Neatness
General neatness of the application or résumé: Is their handwriting readable (consider your records, etc.), résumé typed and error-free?—How is the applicant's spelling and grammar?

Completeness
Completeness on the résumé and application: Did they fill in all the blanks? Is the information on dates, etc., complete?

Experience
Length of experience, type, amount of demonstrated responsibility, types of positions held, etc.

Work History
Do they have a good work record? How long do they stay at each position? What were some of their reasons for leaving?

Education
Do they continue their professional growth through special classes, workshops, special on-the-job training, evening college? Involvement in professional groups or clubs?

How Do They Sell Themselves?
Do they know how to amplify their skills and strengths? How do they demonstrate their level of self-confidence?

Initiative
Do they offer anything besides the basics?

English Skills
Do they use appropriate English in the interview and on the application or résumé?

STAFF SURVEY

Name _____ Position _____ Years with Practice _____

Please circle as appropriate

Salary, for position	1. Below par	2. At par	3. Above par	4. Don't know
Fringe benefits, for position	1. Below par	2. At par	3. Above par	4. Don't know
Staff interrelationships	1. Below par	2. At par	3. Above par	4. Excellent except for 1 or 2 persons
Performance reviews	1. Never or almost never	2. Occasionally	3. Regular	
Duties	1. Not clearly defined	2. Some defined, some not	3. Clearly defined with job descriptions	
Communications	1. Poor—nonconstructive criticism	2. Occasional praise, some helpful criticism	3. Doctors often praise and constructively criticize when deserved; conversation is usually pleasant, two-way	
Workload	1. Way too much or too little!	2. Usually OK	3. Just right—interesting mix of duties	
Hours	1. Poor—too long, out too late	2. Usually OK	3. Fine	
Training	1. Almost nonexistent	2. Adequate	3. Great! Thorough in office training; attend seminars	
Physical environment	1. Poor—depressing	2. Adequate	3. Pleasant	

Comments/Additions/Explanation

_____

_____

What three things need improving in this practice?

1. _____

2. _____

3. _____

Provide this form to your staff one or two times a year.

TELEPHONE SCREENING APPLICANTS

Always telephone interview applicants before scheduling them for a face-to-face interview.

Telephone interviewing procedures/questions for prospective personnel:

First offer an explanation of the position for which you are screening and let them know that this telephone conversation is just the first step in the process. Explain that they may be called for an interview but that at this time you cannot commit to them.

- Tell me about your skills and experience as you see them relating to the position I have just explained to you.
- Tell me about a process or procedure you changed in an office that made things run more smoothly.
- What experience or project have you been involved with that you are most proud of in your career thus far?
- What do you see as your strengths for the job I have described? (Don't settle for "I deal real well with patients"—ask them to be more specific or ask for other strengths.)
- What do you like about yourself the most?
- What would you most like to change about yourself?
- Explain a situation in which you had an idea for a change in procedures for the office and how you presented the possible change to peers or supervisors.
- What was your favorite job so far in your career? What made it special?
- If others who have worked with you could make some statements about you, what would they say?

Be sure you do not face-to-face interview all the people you phone interview. You are doing something wrong if you do. Use the phone as a screening tool to save time. People who cannot handle the phone well spontaneously will most likely not work for a busy office.

Applicant:	Interviewer:
Date:	Job:

4 = needs improvement 3 = fair 2 = OK 1 = excellent	Listens well	
	Intelligent responses	
	Diction	
	Intelligible	
	Cheerful	
	Discreet	
	Vocabulary	
	Call for interview?	

TIME CARD

Pay Period Ending: _____   Employee: _____

Date	In	Out	In	Out	Total Hours

Reg Hrs. _____

O/T Hrs. _____

Total Hrs. _____

Gross Pay _____

FICA _____

Fed W/H _____

State W/H _____

Insurance _____

Net Pay _____

Note: Record reason for any absences daily such as:
        children ill, employee ill, vacation, etc.

Time cards are recommended if you have more than five employees or tardiness problems. Consider a computer program.

WAGE STATEMENT

Wage Statement

Employee: _____
Number: _____
Social Security Number: _____

Period from: _____

PAYMENTS	NO. HOURS	RATE	TOTAL
Regular hours	_____	_____	_____
Overtime hours	_____	_____	_____
Vacation	_____	_____	_____

TOTAL EARNED [ ]

Social Security (FICA): _____
Federal Withholding: _____
State Withholding Tax: _____
Local Withholding Tax: _____

KEEP THIS RECORD OF YOUR EARNINGS

TOTAL DEDUCTIONS [ ]

TOTAL NET PAY [ ]

Wage Statement

Employee: _____
Number: _____
Social Security Number: _____

Period from: _____

PAYMENTS	NO. HOURS	RATE	TOTAL
Regular hours	_____	_____	_____
Overtime hours	_____	_____	_____
Vacation	_____	_____	_____

TOTAL EARNED [ ]

Social Security (FICA): _____
Federal Withholding: _____
State Withholding Tax: _____
Local Withholding Tax: _____

KEEP THIS RECORD OF YOUR EARNINGS

TOTAL DEDUCTIONS [ ]

TOTAL NET PAY [ ]

Wage Statement

Employee: _____
Number: _____
Social Security Number: _____

Period from: _____

PAYMENTS	NO. HOURS	RATE	TOTAL
Regular hours	_____	_____	_____
Overtime hours	_____	_____	_____
Vacation	_____	_____	_____

TOTAL EARNED [ ]

Social Security (FICA): _____
Federal Withholding: _____
State Withholding Tax: _____
Local Withholding Tax: _____

KEEP THIS RECORD OF YOUR EARNINGS

TOTAL DEDUCTIONS [ ]

TOTAL NET PAY [ ]

Wage Statement

Employee: _____
Number: _____
Social Security Number: _____

Period from: _____

PAYMENTS	NO. HOURS	RATE	TOTAL
Regular hours	_____	_____	_____
Overtime hours	_____	_____	_____
Vacation	_____	_____	_____

TOTAL EARNED [ ]

Social Security (FICA): _____
Federal Withholding: _____
State Withholding Tax: _____
Local Withholding Tax: _____

KEEP THIS RECORD OF YOUR EARNINGS

TOTAL DEDUCTIONS [ ]

TOTAL NET PAY [ ]

YEAR-END OR MONTHLY WAGE AND BENEFIT STATEMENT

Employee: _____

Social Security Number: _____

Wages (regular and overtime)	$
Vacation pay	$
Sick pay	$
Sick pay (compensation for unused days)	$
State unemployment taxes paid by practice (SUI & ERR)	$
Federal unemployment taxes paid by practice (FUTA)	$
Social Security taxes contributed to your account (FICA)	$
Workers' compensation	$
Health insurance	$
Bonuses	$
Continuing education	$
Uniform allowances	$
Association dues/professional services	$
Miscellaneous	$
a.	$
b.	$
c.	$
d.	$
Total compensation: Per Year	$
Per Month	$
Per Hour	$

Give this form to each staff person at his or her review. It educates the staff persons about their total compensation packages and makes them less susceptible to other job offers.

EMPL. NO. _____   CARD NO. _____

TIME CARD
(Semi-monthly or two weekly)

Full Name_____   Age _____
                                                        (if under 18)
Address_____   Soc. Sec. No. _____
Pay Period
Starting _____   Ending _____   Rate _____   20____

| Date | REGULAR TIME | | | | Total R.T. | Total O.T. | Daily Totals Emp.Init. | TIME OFF | | |
	In	Out	In	Out				Sick	Vac	PTO
Approved By				Total Time						

EARNINGS

Regular Days worked ___ @ ___	Hrs. ___ @ ___		$
Additional Compensation: Value of Meals, Lodging, Gifts, etc.		AMOUNT	$
Commissions, Fees Bonuses, Sales, etc.		AMOUNT	$
Other (Kind)			$
	TOTAL EARNINGS		$

DEDUCTIONS

Federal With-holding Tax			Insurance	
State With-holding Tax			Other	
Social Security Tax			Cash Advanced	
State Unemploy-ment Ins.				
			TOTAL DEDUCTIONS	$ _____
			NET PAY	$ _____

I certify the foregoing to be a correct account of the time worked and wages received:

                                                        DATE
SIGNATURE _____   **PAID** _____

426

FORM P-20

WEEKLY TIME TICKET

WEEKLY TIME TICKET

EMPLOYEE'S NAME_____ No. _____ Week Ending _____ 20___

Job Name or No	Kind of Work Done	S	M	T	W	T	F	S	Hrs.	Rate	Amount	
	Total Regular Time											
	Total Overtime											
APPROVED BY	WITHHOLD	SDI	FICA		STATE WH				Total Earnings			
									Total Deductions			
	Date Paid		Check No.						NET PAY			

*Systems Forms*_____

Introduction

This section contains forms related to office function, such as scheduling and recall, helpful checklists, and a few forms we couldn't' decide where else to place.

The more you can systemize your practice, the smoother it will flow. When you need a temp to fill in for a sick employee, he or she can more easily step in if there is a written system of who does what and when. Written lists help regular staff remember details. Tracking patient waits gives you data for discussion with the doctors about coming in late. Termination letters help those intolerable patients find better relationships with other providers.

AUTHORIZATION FOR DISCLOSURE OF HIV TEST RESULTS

I hereby authorize _____, M.D., to release the HIV test results

of _____(patient) to _____ .

This authorization is limited to the following purpose: _____

_____

This authorization is effective immediately and shall remain in effect until

_____ (date).

I understand that the requestor may not further use or disclose this medical information unless I authorize such further use or disclosure or unless such use or disclosure is specifically required or permitted by law.

Signed _____ Date _____

If not signed by patient, please indicate relationship:

[ ]   parent or guardian of minor patient under 12 years old
[ ]   guardian or conservator of incompetent patient

AUTHORIZATION FOR RELEASE OF RECORDS PURSUANT TO SUBPOENA

I hereby authorize _____, M.D., to produce the medical records requested in the Deposition Subpoena for Business Records issued _____ (date subpoena issued).

Signed: _____ Date: _____

If not signed by patient, please indicate relationship:

[ ]   attorney representing patient in a lawsuit
[ ]   personal representative of deceased patient
[ ]   parent or guardian of minor patient
[ ]   guardian or conservator of incompetent patient

434

FAMILY PHYSICIAN APPOINTMENT TYPES FOR SCHEDULING

Type	MA time	Dr. time	MA time
Complete H&P/Preop (MA complete forms)			
Precomplete H&P			
Prekindergarten			
DMV			
WELL CHILD EXAM			
2, 4, 5, 15, 18 months with shots			
PROCEDURES			
Flex sig			
Endometrial BX			
Excisional BX (limit to end of am/pm)			
Vasectomy (pm only)			
Norplant/IUD			
Foreign body of eye			
Removal of nail			
Punch BX			
OTHER			
Anxiety/stress (first OV)			
Sore throat, rash, UTI, bruise, ear pain, cough, eye (except injury), fevers age 20 to adult, abd. pain, fatigue			
Follow-up depression			
Headache			
Backache			
Pap only			
Dizziness			
Referral request			
FIVE-MINUTE APPOINTMENT			
Suture removal			
Wound check			
Recheck on UTI, ear, abscess			
IMMEDIATE APPOINTMENT			
Chest pain, baby with fever, asthma, bleeding laceration, vaginal discharge, breast lump			

Provide a list of times for your receptionist. Fill this out together with the whole staff.

GOAL SETTING

Purpose:

Date:

Persons Present:

Page: of:

Goal	Task Involved	Target Date	Who Initials	Anticipated Results	Date Compl

438

MEDICAL RECALL MODEL

APPOINTMENT POSTCARD

It's time for your return appointment

☐ Please call our office to schedule a visit.

☐ Your appointment is scheduled for:

_____

If this is not convenient, please call immediately.

Dr. Name
Address
City, CA ZIP
(123) 456-7890

CONTROL CARD

Name, Last, First _____

Phone _____

Address _____

Notes:

©2003 Professional Management & Marketing

Medical Recall Model

For prevention of "lost patients," control of return visit scheduling, and documentation of follow-up.

This system is designed for those patients coming in less than once a month. Patient needing an appointment sooner should be scheduled into the appointment book and given a reminder call 24 to 48 hours in advance of that appointment.

System:

A 3-by-5 file box with monthly dividers. Enough control cards to callow one per patient in the system. Postcard/appointment reminder cards. Patient chart.

Process:

1. Dr. announces number of months until next appointment.

2. Staff hands patient a postcard to self-address. Use a folding postcard for confidentiality if appropriate. Staff fills out a control card if one does not exist. Staff assigns a return appointment. Staff writes time and date on postcard, control card, appointment book, and patient chart.

3. Put postcard and control card together in month of appointment section of file box (alphabetically). Put the control card upright and the postcard on end so it sticks up.

4. In the last week of the month preceding the appointment, pull all postcards for the upcoming month and mail them.

5. Call the patient the day before his or her appointment to confirm. If the patient is not reached, log activity on control card.

6. When patient comes in and completes appointment, go to 1.

7. At the end of the month, any remaining control cards should reflect patients due but not seen. Process them.

MEDICAL RECORD DOCUMENTATION AUDIT

Year _____ Specialty _____ Dr. _____

Indicator	% Compliance
Alpha tabs	
Annual tabs	
Drug alert tabs	
Sex	
Date of birth	
Home address	
Home or work phone number	
Occupation	
Employer	
Patient name on all pages	
Organized	
Complete problem summary	
Complete Rx summary	
Allergies and adverse reactions	
Entries dated	
Entries initialed	
Legibility	

©2003 Professional Management & Marketing

Audit 100 of your charts annually for compliance.

OFFICE MANAGER CHECKLIST

	Daily	Weekly	Monthly	Quarterly	Semiannually	Annually
Person Responsible: Office Manager Date: _____						
Account receivable—aging review (collections)						
Production goals set and monitored actively						
Billings/production/charges for the month reviewed						
Scheduling "working" and "not working" reviewed						
New patient count/flow						
Referral pattern or new patient source review						
Insurance billing report						
Over-the-counter collections	Spot Check					
Cash flow general						
Accounts to/at collection agency						
Day sheets balance to ledger cards monthly or computer balancing/reports run for month end	Spot Check					
Accounts payable reporting						
Balance checkbook/bank reconciliation						
No. patients on day sheet/computer = no. shown on schedule	Spot Check					
Profit and loss review						
Budget issues						
Auditing—accounting or billing procedures						
Payroll taxes paid/deposited						
Inventory—office supplies medical supplies/medical samples, etc.						
Special projects progress						
Personnel review/report						
Profit center review						
Chart audit	As Needed					
Recall system effectiveness review						
Marketing projects report—internal and external						
Cross-check receipt nos. with pts. shown on ledgers or computer						
Review of management reports from computer/bookkeeper						

Having a schedule like this provides the manager with proper expectations and guidelines. It also helps ensure that something doesn't get missed for too long.

OFFICE REPORT CARD

To help us serve you better, we would appreciate your filling in this report card on our office.

	LOW		HIGH	
Did we greet you promptly and cheerfully?	1	2	3	4
Was our office neat and clean?	1	2	3	4
How is our magazine selection?	1	2	3	4
How do you like our office décor?	1	2	3	4
Was there adequate parking?	1	2	3	4
Were you seen on time?	1	2	3	4
If we were late, was it explained?	1	2	3	4
Have your phone calls or lab results been returned promptly?	1	2	3	4
Do you like being called by your first name?	1	2	3	4
Were you comfortable during your treatment?	1	2	3	4
Was our staff courteous?	1	2	3	4
Have we answered your questions clearly?	1	2	3	4
Did you understand why particular care was recommended?	1	2	3	4
How well are we responding to your needs?	1	2	3	4
Would you recommend us to your family and friends?	1	2	3	4

As a patient of Dr. _____ I would like to tell him/her _____

_____

_____

Additional suggestions that might help us serve you better would be appreciated.

_____

_____

_____

_____

Thank you for your help and cooperation!

Your name below is optional. If you would like a response, please enter your name and phone number.

_____

PATIENT PRIVACY NOTICE REGARDING SUBPOENA

TO _____(patient) AND TO YOUR ATTORNEY OF RECORD:

PLEASE TAKE NOTICE THAT:

(1) RECORDS PERTAINING TO YOU ARE BEING SOUGHT by _____ from _____, M.D., as set forth in the subpoena attached to this Notice.

(2) IF YOU OBJECT to this physician furnishing all or any of the records described in this document to the party seeking such records, YOU MUST FILE PAPERS WITH THE COURT PRIOR TO _____ (date).

(3) YOU OR YOUR ATTORNEY MAY CONTACT the attorney for the party seeking to examine such records to determine whether they are willing to agree IN WRITING to cancel or limit this subpoena. If no such agreement is reached and if you are not otherwise represented by an attorney in this action, YOU SHOULD CONSULT AN ATTORNEY to advise you about your rights or privacy.

Signed: _____   Date: _____

PATIENT REFERRAL LOG

Patient Name Account No.	Referred to (lab, radiology, consultant, etc.)	Date Referred	Date Report Received	Follow-up, by Whom, Date

PROJECT LOG

Name _____

Date in	Date due	Date out	Project Description	Req. by

Keep track and show to your supervisor weekly.

RECOMMENDED TERMINATION LETTER

Letter of Withdrawal from a Case

Dear _____:

I find it necessary to inform you that I am withdrawing from further professional attendance upon you for the reason that you have persisted in refusing to follow my medical advice and treatment. Since your condition requires medical attention, I suggest that you place yourself under the care of another physician without delay. If you so desire, I shall be available to attend you for a reasonable time after you have received this letter, but in no event for more than five days.

This should give you ample time to select a physician of your choice from the many competent physicians in this city. With your approval, I will make available to this physician your case history and information regarding the diagnosis and treatment you have received from me.

Very truly yours,

_____, M.D.

Modify to suit the particular reason. Some practices give two weeks.

RESPONSE TO INVALID DEPOSITION SUBPOENA FOR MEDICAL RECORDS

We received a subpoena on _____ (date) in the case of
_____ (name of case) requesting production of the
medical records of _____ (patient). This subpoena
does not comply with the following requirement(s):

[ ]　The subpoena was not personally served.

[ ]　The subpoena was not accompanied by the required proof of service on or written
authorization from the patient.

[ ]　The subpoena was not served on the patient in a timely manner before it was served on us.

[ ]　The subpoena required the production of records with inadequate time after the subpoena was
issued.

[ ]　The subpoena required the production of records with inadequate time after the subpoena was
served on us.

[ ]　Other: _____
_____
_____

We may not release a patient's medical records in response to an invalid subpoena. I have returned
the subpoena (and retained a file copy for our records) so that you may correct these problems.

Please don't hesitate to call if you have any questions about this letter.

Sincerely,

STAFF POSITION CHECKLIST

	Daily	Weekly	Monthly	Quarterly	Semiannually	Annually
Person Responsible: _____ Date: _____						

458

TASK ANALYSIS CHECKLIST

Staff Name: _____ Date: _____						
Answer the telephone						
Schedule patient appointments						
Maintain listing of telephone callback						
Check for messages with the answering service						
Dial outgoing calls for doctor						
Telephone pharmacists						
Return nonemergency calls for doctors						
Receive patients						
Register patient arrival						
Communicate with "no-show" patients						
Schedule detail rep. appointments						
Schedule appointments with accounts						
Prepare "thank yous" to referring patients						
Maintain doctor's personal appointment log						
Verify new patient credit information						
Prepare a daily work schedule (patient appointments)						
Conduct daily work schedule staff meeting						
Maintain laundry supply records						
Maintain equipment maintenance schedule						
Maintain patient recall, reminder file						
Maintain "periodic" task reminder file						
Open the office						
Make coffee						
Open, sort, and distribute mail						
Order needed janitorial services						
Do office housekeeping chores						
Quiet noisy children						
Renew magazine subscriptions						
Pull records for tomorrow's patients						
Check lab cases for tomorrow's patients						
Confirm appointments for tomorrow						
Inventory and originate order for professional supplies						
Conduct office staff training in new procedures						
Schedule and conduct regular staff meetings						
Post charges and payments						
Post payments received in mail						
Prepare and mail monthly statements						
Follow up on delinquent accounts with doctor; take action						
Prepare management reports for doctor and accountant						
Review management reports with doctor						
Send necessary materials to accountant's office						

Things go more smoothly when everyone knows who is primarily responsible for what. You can always cross-cover and help each other out too.

TASK ANALYSIS CHECKLIST

Staff name: _____ Date: _____						
Prepare and mail insurance claims on a daily basis						
File claim forms in suspense file until payment received						
Follow up control procedure on old claims						
Telephone insurance company about unpaid claims						
Post payments for insurance company to patient ledger						
Dispose difference between pt. bill and ins. co. reimbursement						
Endorse checks received from patients						
Handle disposition of patient "rubber checks"						
Prepare checks for overpayment to the order of patient						
Determine correcting entries needed in patient ledger						
Prepare patient ledger adjustment forms						
Maintain and replenish petty cash fund						
Check invoices from suppliers for discounts						
Prepare checks for doctor's signature						
Review and sign expense checks						
Record disbursement in daily journal						
Record all cash received in daily journal						
Prepare bank deposit						
Make bank deposit and obtain receipt						
Reconcile the bank balance						
Run a trial balance of accounts						
Prepare payroll checks						
Sign payroll checks						
Record payroll disbursement in ledger						
Deposit payroll withholding tax with bank						
Maintain a listing of office problems						
Schedule and assign unusual tasks						
Take corrective action on an employee problem						
Conduct a salary review						
Compose patient medical correspondence						
Medical—legal scheduling						
Medical—legal paperwork/requests for records						
Type and prepare correspondence						
Keep exam rooms stocked with supplies						
Distribute schedules to various locations						
Make sure instruments are sterilized and trays set up						
Charting procedures and treatment plans prepared						
Enter each procedure on superbill for front desk						
Give postop instructions						
Take x-rays						
Check patient's medical history for health problems						
Escort patient to exam room						

Thank You

for referring

your friends

and family

Copy onto colored paper, frame, and hang in appropriate locations.

WAIT TIME TRACKING

Patient Name	Arrival Time	Appointment Time	Time Seen by Doctor	Wait from Appointment Time to Time Seen
1				
2				
3				
4				
5				
6				
7				
8				
9				
10				
11				
12				
13				
14				
15				
16				
17				
18				
19				
20				
21				
22				
23				
24				

Average number of early arrivals: _____   Longest wait of the day: _____

Average number of late arrivals: _____   Shortest wait of the day: _____

Daily average wait: _____

WEEKLY SCHEDULE

	Monday	Tuesday	Wednesday	Thursday	Friday	Saturday
7:00						
7:30						
8:00						
8:30						
9:00						
9:30						
10:00						
10:30						
11:00						
11:30						
12:00						
12:30						
1:00						
1:30						
2:00						
2:30						
3:00						
3:30						
4:00						
4:30						
5:00						
5:30						
6:00						
6:30						

Use for staff scheduling, multidoctor summary, who washes the coffee cups and when, or patient scheduling in a very laid back practice.

WILL CALL LIST

Patients to be called and rescheduled, including all cancellations, no-shows, patients wanting to be seen sooner, and scheduled patients with flexible schedules that can be moved.

Name Last Name First	Date	New Apt. Date	New Apt. Time	Notes

WORK/SCHOOL RELEASE

WORK/SCHOOL RELEASE

TO: _____

FROM: _____

REPORT DATE: _____

This is to verify that _____

who is currently under my care:

Was seen in my office on _____

☐　　Is to remain off/out of work/school until _____

☐　　Patient can return to work/school as of: _____

☐　　Upon return to work, level of activity should be:

　　☐　　Light duty

　　☐　　Normal duty

☐　　Is to be excused from P.E. class until: _____

☐　　Can return to regular P.E. class if: _____

☐　　May participate in P.E. class limited to: _____

Comments: _____

_____

_____

If you should have any questions or concerns regarding the above information or if we can be of further assistance to you, please feel free to contact our office.

Software and Information License

The software and information on this disk (collectively referred to as the "Product") are the property of PRACTICE MANAGEMENT INFORMATION CORPORATION ("PMIC") and are protected by both United States copyright law and international copyright treaty provision. You must treat this Product just like a book, except that you may copy it into a computer to be used and you may make archival copies of the Product for the sole purpose of backing up our software and protecting your investment from loss.

By saying, "just like a book" PMIC means, for example, that the Product may be used by any number of people and may be freely moved from one computer location to another, so long as there is no possibility that the Product (or any part of the Product) will be used at one location or on one computer while it is being used at another. Just as a book cannot be read by two different people in two different places at the same time (unless, of course, PMIC's rights are being violated).

PMIC reserves the right to alter or modify the contents of the Product at any time.

This Agreement is effective until terminated. The Agreement will terminate automatically without notice if you fail to comply with any provisions of this Agreement. In the event of termination by reason of your breach, you will destroy or erase all copies of the Product installed on any computer system or made for backup purposes and shall expunge the Product from your data storage facilities.

Limited Warranty

PMIC warrants the physical software enclosed herein to be free of defects in materials and workmanship for a period of sixty days from the purchase date. If PMIC receives written notification within the warranty period of defects in materials or workmanship, and if such notification is determined by PMIC to be correct, PMIC will replace the defective disk(s). Send Request to:

Practice Management Information Corp.
4727 Wilshire Blvd. 1st Floor Receiving
Los Angeles, CA 90010
Attn: Returns

The entire and exclusive liability and remedy for breach of this Limited Warranty shall be limited to replacement of defective disk(s) and shall not include or extend to any claim for or right to cover any damages, including but not limited to, loss of profit, data, or use of the software, or special, incidental, or consequential damages or other similar claims, even if PMIC has been specifically advised as to the possibility of such damages. In no event will PMIC's liability for any damages to you or any other person ever exceed the lower of suggested list price or actual price paid for the license to use the Product, regardless of any form of the claim.

PMIC specifically disclaims all other warranties, express or implied, including but not limited to, any implied warrant of merchantability or fitness for a particular purpose. Specifically, PMIC makes no representation or warranty that the product is fit for any particular purpose and any implied warranty of merchantability is limited to the sixty day duration of the Limited Warranty covering the physical disk(s) only (and not the software or information) and is otherwise specifically disclaimed.

This limited Warranty gives you specific legal rights; you may have others which may vary from state to state. Some states do not allow the exclusion of incidental or consequential damages, or the limitation on how long an implied warranty lasts, so some of the above may not apply to you.

This Agreement constitutes the entire agreement between the parties relating to use of the Product. The terms of any purchase order shall have no effect on the terms of this Agreement. Failure of PMIC to insist any time on strict compliance with this Agreement shall not constitute a waiver of any rights under this Agreement. This Agreement shall be construed and governed in accordance with the laws of California. In any provision of this Agreement is held to be contrary to law, that provision will be enforced to the maximum extent permissible and the remaining provisions will remain in force and effect.